121 Complete Weight Gaining Shake and Meal Recipes to Get Bigger and Stronger:

Meal and Shake Recipes That Will Help You Gain Weight Faster

By

Joe Correa CSN

COPYRIGHT

© 2017 Live Stronger Faster Inc.

This publication is designed to provide accurate and authoritative information in regard to the subject matter covered. It is sold with the understanding that neither the author nor the publisher is engaged in rendering medical advice. If medical advice or assistance is needed, consult with a doctor. This book is considered a guide and should not be used in any way detrimental to your health. Consult with a physician before starting this nutritional plan to make sure it's right for you.

ACKNOWLEDGEMENTS

This book is dedicated to all the people in the world that have had mild or serious illnesses so that you may find a solution and make the necessary changes in your life.

121 Complete Weight Gaining Shake and Meal Recipes to Get Bigger and Stronger:

Meal and Shake Recipes That Will Help You Gain Weight Faster

By

Joe Correa CSN

CONTENTS

ABOUT THE AUTHOR

After years of Research, I honestly believe in the positive effects that proper nutrition can have over the body and mind. My knowledge and experience has helped me live healthier throughout the years and which I have shared with family and friends. The more you know about eating and drinking healthier, the sooner you will want to change your life and eating habits.

Nutrition is a key part in the process of being healthy and living longer so get started today. The first step is the most important and the most significant.

INTRODUCTION

121 Complete Weight Gaining Shake and Meal Recipes to Get Bigger and Stronger: Meal and Shake Recipes That Will Help You Gain Weight Faster

By Joe Correa CSN

Gaining weight can be difficult and will require hard work. These shake, juice, and meal recipes will help you organize what you eat so that you can do it in a healthy and consistent manner. Make your life easier by knowing what to eat.

Whether your condition is clinically defined as underweight, or you simply want to gain some muscles, your new lifestyle will be the same. The most important component of the weight gaining process is definitely proper nutrition. Now you might think that the easiest way to do this would be to simply increase the number of burgers and pizzas you eat every day, but unfortunately, that's not the case. Just like with obesity, gaining weight requires some healthy nutrients that your body will actually use. Your daily menu must have a good amount of healthy fats, good carbs, and precious proteins.

Healthy fats like omega-3 fatty acids can be found in fatty fish like salmon, fish oil, olives, olive oil, chia seeds, walnuts, and spinach. One serving of wild salmon fillet, for example, is probably the best way to eat some good fats and gain some controlled weight. Lean beef, fish, poultry, legumes, and nuts should be your number one choice of proteins. Eat at least three servings of these foods per day. Regarding carbs, you should choose fruits, vegetables, and whole grains. This formula is proven not only to give you an ideal weight but also to improve your overall health in an amazing and tasty way.

Resistance and strength training have been proven to increase muscle mass and should be incorporated in your daily routine.

Combine excellent nutrition with resistance and strength training using these powerful weight gaining recipes to make a real change. Start now and see the results in no time!

121 COMPLETE WEIGHT GAINING SHAKE AND MEAL RECIPES TO GET BIGGER AND STRONGER: MEAL AND SHAKE RECIPES THAT WILL HELP YOU GAIN WEIGHT FASTER

MEALS

1.　Penne Pasta with Shrimp

Ingredients:

1 lb of penne pasta, pre-cooked

1 lb of shrimps, peeled and deveined

1 cup of Greek yogurt

1 cup of tomatoes, diced

2 tbsp of tomato paste

1 cup of celery, chopped

1 cup of green onions, chopped

1 tsp of fresh rosemary, finely chopped

1 tbsp of fresh parsley, finely chopped

½ tsp of sea salt

¼ tsp of black pepper, ground

Preparation:

Cook pasta using package instructions. Remove from the heat and drain well. Set aside.

Combine tomatoes, tomato paste, rosemary, parsley, salt, and pepper in a medium bowl. Mix well and set aside.

Place green onions and celery in a large nonstick saucepan over a medium-high temperature. Cook for 2 minutes and add shrimps. Add 1 cup of water and cook for 15 minutes, or until shrimps are tender. Stir in the tomato mixture. Cook for 3 minutes, or until thickens. Stir in the pasta and cook for 2 minutes more, stirring constantly. Remove from the heat and add yogurt. Stir well and serve immediately.

Nutritional information per serving: Kcal: 350, Protein: 29.8g, Carbs: 47.9g, Fats: 3.8g

2.   Southern Chicken

Ingredients:

1 lb of chicken breasts, skinless and boneless

4 tbsp of tomato paste

2 tsp of honey, raw

2 garlic cloves, minced

1 small onion, diced

1 tsp of Worcestershire sauce

4 tsp of white wine vinegar

¼ tsp of Cayenne pepper, ground

¼ tsp of black pepper, ground

¼ tsp of ginger, ground

½ tsp of salt

Preparation:

Preheat the oven to 375°F.

Combine tomato paste, honey, garlic, onion, Worcestershire sauce, vinegar, cayenne pepper, pepper, ginger, and salt in a large saucepan over a medium-high temperature. Cook for 15 minutes, stirring constantly. Remove from the heat and set aside.

Wash and pat dry the meat. Place the meat on a large baking sheet and add about half of the previously prepared sauce. You can use kitchen brush, or simply pour over. Cover with a plastic wrap and refrigerate at least for 1 hour.

Now, replace the plastic wrap with aluminum foil and place it in the oven. Bake for 10 minutes on each side. Reduce the heat to 350°F and add remaining sauce. Bake for another 30 minutes.

Remove from the oven and serve immediately.

Nutritional information per serving: Kcal: 336, Protein: 45.1g, Carbs: 11.4g, Fats: 11.4g

3.   Choco-Coco Smoothie

Ingredients:

1 large egg

1 tbsp of coconut oil

1 tsp of chia seeds

¼ cup coconut milk

½ cup of water

1 tsp of stevia

1 tbsp of raw cocoa, sugar-free

½ tsp of vanilla extract, sugar-free

Preparation:

Place the ingredients in a blender and pulse to combine. Serve cold.

Nutritional information per serving: Kcal: 393 , Protein: 12.7g, Carbs: 18.2, Fats: 41.3g

4.   Pizza Stuffed Peppers

Ingredients:

3 large green bell peppers

2 large tomatoes, roughly chopped

2 tbsp of tomato pizza sauce, sugar-free

1 tsp of dried oregano

½ tsp of thyme

4oz mozzarella cheese sliced

3 tbsp of parmesan cheese

1 tbsp parsley, finely chopped

4 tbsp of extra virgin olive oil

½ tsp of salt

¼ tsp of freshly ground black pepper

Preparation:

Preheat the oven to 350 degrees. Line some baking paper over a baking sheet and set aside.

Using a sharp knife, cut the peppers in half and remove the seeds. Grease each papper inside with some olive oil. Set aside.

In a medium-sized bowl, combine mozzarella with tomatoes, pizza tomato sauce, thyme, oregano, parsley, and two tablespoons of olive oil. Stir well and use the mixture to stuff each pepper half. Add some salt and pepper and top with parmesan.

Bake for 20 minutes.

Nutrition information per serving: Kcal: 205, Protein: 11g, Carbs: 5g, Fats: 12g

5.   Trout Stew with Potatoes

Ingredients:

1 lb of trout fillets, cleaned

4 medium-sized potatoes, peeled and chopped

1 cup of tomatoes, diced

2 small onions, chopped

3 garlic cloves, finely chopped

½ cup of spring onions, chopped

½ tsp of chili pepper, ground

½ tsp of vegetable seasoning mix

½ tsp of salt

½ tsp of black pepper, ground

Preparation:

Combine potatoes, tomatoes, garlic, and onions in a large saucepan. Pour water enough to cover all ingredients and bring it to a boil over a medium-high temperature. Cook for 15 minutes, then reduce the heat to medium-low. Cook for another 15 minutes then add fish fillets. Sprinkle with chili, vegetable seasoning mix, and black pepper. Cover with a lid and cook for the next 20 minutes.

Meanwhile, preheat the oil in a large frying pan over a medium-high temperature. Add fillets and sprinkle with rosemary. Fry for 5 minutes on each side, or until set. Remove from the heat and set aside to cool for a while. Chop the fish into bite-sized pieces and add to the pot with vegetables. Cook for 10 minutes more and remove from the heat.

Garnish with spring onions before serving.

Nutritional information per serving: Kcal: 225, Protein: 20.0g, Carbs: 23.1g, Fats: 5.7g

6.   Turkey with Green Beans

Ingredients:

1 lb of turkey breasts, skinless and boneless

1 lb of green beans, cut into bite-sized pieces

1 medium onion, finely chopped

2 tbsp of fresh parsley, finely chopped

3 tbsp of olive oil

½ tsp of salt

¼ tsp of black pepper, ground

Preparation:

Place the beans in a pot of boiling water and cook for about 10-12 minutes, or until fork tender. Remove from the heat and drain well.

Preheat 2 tablespoons of oil in a large frying pan over a medium-high temperature. Cook for 5 minutes on each side, or until golden brown. Remove from the heat and set aside, but reserve the pan.

Add the remaining oil and onion. Stir-fry for 5 minutes, or until translucent. Add green beans and sprinkle with some salt and pepper to taste. Cook until heated through. Remove from the heat and transfer to a serving plate with meat. Sprinkle with parsley and serve immediately.

Nutritional information per serving: Kcal: 204, Protein: 17.4g, Carbs: 12.5g, Fats: 10.1g

7.   Choco Walnut Smoothie

Ingredients:

½ cup of walnuts, chopped

1 cup of Greek yogurt

¼ cup of chocolate chips

1 large banana, chopped

2 tbsp of flaxseeds

Preparation:

Combine all ingredients in a food processor and blend until nicely smooth. Transfer to a serving glasses and refrigerate for 1 hour before serving.

Nutritional information per serving: Kcal: 473, Protein: 20.5g, Carbs: 36.8g, Fats: 28.9g

8.   Maccaroni & Cheese

Ingredients:

3 cups of maccaroni

1 cup of Cheddar cheese, shredded

1 large egg

1 cup of sour cream

1 medium-sized onion, finely chopped

¼ tsp of black pepper, ground

Preparation:

Preheat the oven to 350°F.

Cook maccaroni using package instructions, but without salt. Drain well and set aside.

Combine maccaroni, cheese and egg in a large bowl. Set aside.

Grease a baking sheet or a casserole dish with some cooking spray. Add onions and cook for 3-4 minutes on a medium-high temperature. remove from the heat and add maccaroni mixture. Place it in the oven and bake for 25 minutes, or until bubbly. Remove from the heat and stir in the sour cream.

Sprinkle with some extra cheese and serve.

Nutritional information per serving: Kcal: 482, Protein: 19.2g, Carbs: 46.6g, Fats: 24.4g

9.   Potato Omelet

Ingredients:

2 medium-sized potatoes, peeled and chopped

4 large eggs, beaten

1 tbsp of parsley, finely chopped

2 tbsp of Gouda cheese, shredded

1 large bell pepper, chopped

1 small onion, chopped

½ tsp of Himalayan salt

1 tbsp of butter

¼ tsp of black pepper, ground

Preparation:

Place the potatoes in a pot of boiling water and cook until fork-tender. Remove from the heat and drain. Set aside.

Whisk the eggs, salt, and pepper in a mixing bowl. Set aside.

Melt the butter in a frying pan over a medium-high temperature. Add onion, potatoes, and bell pepper. Cook for 5 minutes and then pour the egg mixture. Sprinkle with cheese and cook for 3-4 minutes on each side. Remove from the heat and fold the omelet. Serve immediately.

Nutritional information per serving: Kcal: 232, Protein: 11.8g, Carbs: 21.4g, Fats: 11.5g

10.   Creamy Chicken Soup

Ingredients:

10 oz chicken fillets, cut into bite-sized pieces

1 cup of heavy cream

½ cup of broccoli, chopped

3 cups of chicken stock

1 small zucchini, chopped

2 tbsp of olive oil

1 tbsp of fresh parsley, finely chopped

½ tsp of salt

¼ tsp of black pepper, ground

Preparation:

Melt the butter in a frying pan over a medium-high temperature. Add chicken and cook for 3-4 minutes, or until golden brown. Remove from the heat and set aside.

Combine oil and vegetable stock in a heavy-bottomed pot. Sprinkle with salt and pepper and add broccoli and zucchini. Bring it to a boil and then reduce the heat to medium-low. Cover with a lid and cook for 15 minutes.

Now, remove the vegetables from the pot and transfer to a food processor. Reserve the liquid. Blend until nicely smooth the return to the pot. Add chicken and heavy cream and cook for 10 more minutes. Remove from the heat and garnish with parsley.

Nutritional information per serving: Kcal: 252, Protein: 17.9g, Carbs: 2.6g, Fats: 19.1g

11.   White Meatballs

Ingredients:

1 lb of lean beef, ground

½ cup fo Feta cheese, crumbled

2 large eggs

½ cup of olives, pitted, chopped

4 tbsp of fresh parsley, finely chopped

1 tsp of dried oregano, ground

¼ tsp of black pepper, ground

Preparation:

Combine all ingredients except the oil in a large bowl. Mix with hands and shape the balls. Set aside.

Preheat the oil in a large nonstick skillet over a medium-high temperature. Add meatballs and fry for 10 minutes, or until browned. Remove from the heat and transfer to a serving plate. Pour over the yogurt and serve immediately.

Nutritional information per serving: Kcal: 424, Protein: 54.0g, Carbs: 3.4g, Fats: 20.5g

12.   Grilled Pepper and Tomato Omelet

Ingredients:

1 medium-sized red bell pepper, sliced

1 ripe tomato

2 eggs

1 tbsp of olive oil

Salt and pepper to taste

Dry oregano

Preparation:

Slice the pepper and tomato into thin slices. Heat up the olive oil over medium-high temperature and add the vegetables and oregano. Stir-fry for about 5 minutes, or until lightly charred. Remove from the heat and set aside.

Crack the eggs and beat well with a fork. Season with some salt, pepper and oregano. Fry the eggs for two minutes on each side and transfer to a plate.

Place the vegetables on one-half of the omelet and fold in half.

Nutrition information per serving: Kcal: 268, Protein: 21, Carbs: 4.6g, Fats: 4.7g

13.   Creamy Spinach Omelet

Ingredients:

0.5 lb of fresh spinach, finely chopped

1 cup of kefir (can be replaced with yogurt)

3 tbsp of olive oil

2 whole eggs

Salt to taste

3 tbsp grated Ricotta goat's cheese

Preparation:

Combine the spinach with kefir in a food processor. Mix well for about 20-30 seconds, until smooth mixture.

Heat up the olive oil in a large skillet, over a medium temperature. Pour in the spinach mixture and reduce the heat to minimum. Cook for about 10 minutes and then increase the heat to maximum. Stir-fry for 3-4 minutes and remove from the heat.

Meanwhile, beat the eggs and pour into a frying pan. Add some salt and fry for about a minute on each side. Transfer to a plate, add spinach mixture and fold it over in half.

Sprinkle with grated Ricotta and serve.

Nutrition information per serving: Kcal: 121, Protein: 9g, Carbs: 3g, Fats: 9.1g

14.   Baked Avocado Eggs with Rosemary

Ingredients:

3 medium-sized ripe avocados, cut in half

6 whole eggs

1 medium-sized tomato, finely chopped

3 tbsp of olive oil

2 tsp of dried rosemary

salt and pepper to taste

Preparation:

Preheat oven to 350 degrees. Cut avocado in half and remove the flesh from the center. Place one egg and chopped tomato in each avocado half and sprinkle with rosemary, salt and pepper. Grease the baking pan with olive oil and place the avocados. You want to use a small baking pan so your avocados can fit tightly. Place in the oven for about 15-20 minutes.

Nutrition information per serving: Kcal: 280 Protein: 28g, Carbs: 41g, Fats: 20g

15.   Pesto Kalamata Muffins

Ingredients:

3.5oz fresh spinach, finely chopped

1 medium-sized tomato, finely chopped

4 large eggs

¼ cup of Kalamata olives, pitted and halved

½ cup of fresh goat's cheese, shredded

3 tbsp organic pesto

1 tsp of salt

¼ tsp of freshly ground red pepper

Preparation:

Preheat the oven to 350 degrees. Line one 6-cup muffin tins with paper liners.

Combine finely chopped tomatoes with kalamata, goat's cheese, pesto, salt, and pepper in a large bowl. Gently whisk in the eggs, one at the time, and beat well on high. Continue beating until well incorporated.

Using a spoon or ice cream scoop, divide the mixture evenly among the tins. Bake for 20-30 or until the toothpick inserted into the middle comes out clean.

Let it cool for another 30 minutes.

Nutrition information per serving: Kcal: 110 Protein: 4.8g, Carbs: 1.5g, Fats: 8g

16.   Creamy Brussel Sprouts

Ingredients:

1 lb of Brussel Sprouts, trimmed and halved

¼ cup of cream cheese

5 tbsp of almonds, roughly chopped

½ tsp of sea salt

1 tbsp olive oil

¼ tsp of black pepper, ground

¼ tsp of nutmeg, ground

Preparation:

Place the Brussel sprouts in a pot of boiling water. Cook until tender and remove from the heat. Drain well and return to the pot.Add olive oil and cook for 5 minutes. Add cheese and sprinkle with nutmeg, salt, and pepper to taste. Heat it up and remove from the heat. Sprinkle with almonds before serving.

Nutritional information per serving: Kcal: 231, Protein: 8.7g, Carbs: 16.6g, Fats: 17.0g

17. Mustard Turkey with Asparagus

Ingredients:

1 lb of turkey fillets, skinless and boneless

1 tbsp of butter

2 cups of asparagus

1 cup of chicken broth

2 tbsp of yellow mustard

2 tbsp of olive oil

1 tbsp of fresh parsley, chopped

½ tsp of salt

1 cup of water

Preparation:

Rub the salt, pepper, and garlic into the fillets and set aside for 10 minutes.

Place the asparagus into a pot of boiling water. Cook until tender and remove from the heat. Drain well and set aside.

Melt the butter in a large skillet over a medium-high temperature. Place the fillets and cook for 4-5 minutes on each side, or until golden brown. Add broth and reduce the heat to low. Bring it to a boil and remove from the heat.

Combine oil, mustard, parsley, and salt in a mixing bowl. Drain the liquid from the skillet to the mixing bowl and stir in with mustard. Place the fillets on a serving plate and serve with asparagus. Pour over the sauce and serve immediately.

Nutritional information per serving: Kcal: 245, Protein: 29.0g, Carbs: 2.6g, Fats: 13.0g

18.   Spaghetti Mussels

Ingredients:

1 lb of mussels, with shells

1 lb of spaghetti pasta, pre-cooked

4 garlic cloves, finely chopped

4 tbsp butter

1 cup of chicken broth

1 medium-sized onion, finely chopped

4 tbsp of apple juice, freshly squeezed

3 tbsp of parsley, finely chopped

2 bay leaves

Preparation:

Cook the pasta using package instructions. Remove from the heat and drain well. Set aside.

Wash the mussels and remove all with any damages or cracks.

Combine garlic, chicken broth, onion, and apple juice in a large skillet over a medium-high temperature. Bring it to a boil and add bay leaves. Now, reduce the heat to medium-low and cover with a lid. Add the mussels and cook for 5-6 minutes, stirring or shaking the skillet.

In a medium frying pan, melt the butter and add parsley. Stir well and remove from the heat.

Serve the pasta on a serving plate, and top with mussels. Drizzle with butter and sprinkle with some extra salt and pepper to taste, if needed.

Nutritional information per serving: Kcal: 380, Protein: 16.2g, Carbs: 56.1g, Fats: 9.9g

19.   Avocado Pasta

Ingredients:

1 lb of rotini pasta, pre-cooked

1 medium-sized avocado, pitted and peeled

2 small tomatoes, diced

1 celery stalk, chopped

2 tbsp of fresh parsley, finely chopped

2 tsp of lemon juice, freshly squeezed

For the dressing:

1 medium-sized avocado, pitted and peeled

4 tbsp of lemon juice, freshly squeezed

½ tsp of cumin, ground

1 cup of Greek yogurt

½ tsp of salt

½ tsp of black pepper, ground

Preparation:

Cook the pasta using package instructions. Sprinkle with some salt while cooking. Remove from the heat and drain well. Set aside.

In a large bowl, combine chopped avocado, tomatoes, celery, parsley, and lemon juice. Stir in the pasta and aside.

Combine all dressing ingredients in a food processor and blend until creamy and smooth. Drizzle with avocado sauce and refrigerate for at least 1 hour.

Enjoy!

Nutritional information per serving: Kcal: 466, Protein: 16.1g, Carbs: 60.2g, Fats: 18.8g

20.   Beef and Veggies Bake

Ingredients:

1 lb of lean beef, cut into bite-sized pieces

1 cup of button mushrooms, chopped

2 large potatoes, peeled and sliced

1 cup of sour cream

¼ cup of spring onions, chopped

3 garlic cloves, crushed

2 small carrots, sliced

4 tbsp of olive oil

1 tbsp of butter

1 tbsp of Dijon mustard

½ tsp of salt

½ tsp of black pepper, ground

2 bay leaves

Preparation:

Preheat the oven to 400°F.

Coat the meat with mustard and set aside.

Slice the potatoes and spread evenly on a lightly greased baking dish.

Preheat the oil in a large skillet over a medium-high temperature. Add spring onions and carrots. Cook for 3 minutes, then add garlic. Cook for another 2 minutes, or until slightly tender. Remove from the heat and transfer to a baking dish with potatoes. Reserve the pan.

Melt the butter in the same pan over a medium-high temperature. Add the meat and cook for 3 minutes, stirring constantly. Add mushrooms and cook for 10 more minutes, or until golden brown. Transfer all to a baking dish with vegetables. Top with sour cream and 1 cup of water. Sprinkle with salt and pepper and place it in the oven. Bake for 1 hour, or until set. Add more water if needed while baking.

Serve warm.

Nutritional information per serving: Kcal: 360, Protein: 23.2g, Carbs: 20.6g, Fats: 20.8g

21.   Avocado Kale Smoothie

Ingredients:

1 ripe avocado, pitted and peeled

1 cup of fresh kale, roughly chopped

1 large banana, chopped

1 cup of Greek yogurt

2 tbsp of flaxseeds

1 tsp of orange zest, for garnish

Preparation:

Combine all ingredients in a food processor and blend until nicely smooth and creamy. Transfer to a serving glasses and refrigerate for 1 hour before serving. Garnish with orange zest.

Nutritional information per serving: Kcal: 259, Protein: 9.5g, Carbs: 22.3g, Fats: 15.9g

22.   Gouda Muffins

Ingredients:

1 cup of Gouda cheese, shredded

4 large eggs

1 cup of fresh spinach, chopped

1 can of tuna, with oil

6 oz of tuna, minced

1 tbsp of parsley, finely chopped

1 tbsp of butter

1 tsp of sea salt

Preparation:

Preheat the oven to 375°F.

Melt the butter in a frying pan over a medium-high temperature. Add spinach and cook for 5 minutes, or until tender. Remove from the heat and add to a large bowl.

Add tuna, cheese, and parsley. Sprinkle with some salt and pepper and mix well using hands. In a lightly greased muffin mold, spoon this mixture. Top with eggs and place it in the oven. Bake for 20 minutes or until set. Remove from the oven and let it cool for a while. Top with extra cheese.

Nutritional information per serving: Kcal: 561, Protein: 54.5g, Carbs: 2.3g, Fats: 36.3g

23.   Tagliatelle Marinara

Ingredients:

1 lb of tagliatelle pasta

1 cup of tomatoes, diced

4 tbsp of tomato paste

4 tbsp of olive oil

1 cup of fresh basil, chopped

1 shallot, chopped

3 garlic cloves, minced

½ tsp of salt

1 tsp of dried oregano, ground

½ tsp of black pepper, ground

Preparation:

Combine tomatoes, tomato paste, basil, shallot, garlic, salt, and pepper in a food processor. Blend for 1 minute, and gradually add oil and re-blend until well incorporated. Set aside

Cook pasta according to a package instructions. Drain well and transfer to a large bowl. Add previously blended mixture and toss well to coat. Sprinkle with oregano and serve immediately.

Nutritional information per serving: Kcal: 476, Protein: 14.4g, Carbs: 68.6g, Fats: 16.9g

24.   Orange Oatmeal

Ingredients:

1 cup of rolled oats

½ cup of plain yogurt

½ cup of water

2 tbsp of dark chocolate, shredded

1 large orange, chopped

2 tbsp of flaxseeds

Preparation:

Combine yogurt, water, and flaxseeds in a mixing bowl. Add oats and stir all well to combine. Top with orange and sprinkle with dark chocolate. Refrigerate or serve immediately!

Nutritional information per serving: Kcal: 335, Protein: 11.8g, Carbs: 51.1g, Fats: 8.8g

25.   Veal Skewers with Sweet Potatoes

Ingredients:

2 lbs of veal shoulder

2 medium-sized sweet potatoes, peeled and chopped

½ cup of olive oil

2 lemons, juiced

2 tbsp of red wine vinegar

4 tbsp of mint, finely chopped

1 tbsp of fresh oregano, minced

1 tsp of salt

½ tsp of black pepper, ground

2 tbsp of sesame seeds

Preparation:

Place the sweet potatoes in a pot of boiling water. Cook until fork-tender and remove from the heat. Drain well and set aside.

Combine oil, mint, oregano, vinegar, salt and pepper in a large bowl. Stir well to mix and set aside to allow flavors to blend.

Dice the meat and soak in the marinade for at least 2 hours.

Preheat the grill to a medium-high temperature. Use metal skewers to arrange the meat and place it on the grill. Reserve the marinade. Grill for 5 minutes on each side, or until golden brown.

Place the skewers and potatoes to a serving plate. Drizzle the potatoes with reserved marinade and sprinkle with sesame seeds before serving.

Nutritional information per serving: Kcal: 490, Protein: 38.5g, Carbs: 16g, Fats: 30g

26.   Sweet Avocado Salad

Ingredients:

1 ripe avocado, pitted, peeled, and chopped

½ cup of strawberries, chopped

2 cups of fresh spinach, chopped

½ cup of cantaloupe, peeled and chopped

1 cup of heavy cream

¼ cup of honey

2 tbsp of balsamic vinegar

1 tbsp of olive oil

½ tsp of salt

½ tsp of black pepper, ground

Preparation:

Combine honey, heavy cream, vinegar, oil, salt and pepper in a mixing bowl. Stir well to mix and set aside to allow flavors to mingle.

In a large salad bowl, combine avocado, strawberries, spinach, and cantaloupe. Stir once, then drizzle with the dressing. Toss well to coat and refrigerate for 30 minutes before serving.

Nutritional information per serving: Kcal: 425, Protein: 3.2g, Carbs: 35.2g, Fats: 32.8g

27.   Breakfast Creamy Mozzarella Tricolore

Ingredients:

2 large tomatoes, sliced

3.5oz mozzarella, sliced

1 medium-sized avocado, halved and stone removed

3 tbsp of extra virgin olive oil

½ tsp of salt

1 tsp of apple cider vinegar

½ tsp of dried thyme, crushed

½ tsp of sugar

Preparation:

Wash and slice tomatoes. Place them on a serving platter.

Cut avocado in half and remove the stone. Slice thinly and make a layer over tomatoes. Top with mozzarella.

In a small bowl, whisk together olive oil, apple cider, thyme, salt, and sugar. Drizzle over tricolore and serve.

Nutrition information per serving: Kcal: 340 Protein: 16.5g, Carbs: 5.8g, Fats: 31g

28.   Sweet Cashew and Raspberry Smoothie

Ingredients:

1 cup of cashew milk

1 whole egg

1 tbsp of raw cocoa

3.5oz avocado, roughly chopped

1 tsp of sugar

1 tsp of raspberry extract

1 tbsp of walnuts, minced

Preparation:

Place the ingredients in a blender and pulse until smooth mixture. Serve cold.

Nutrition information per serving: Kcal: 280 Protein: 16.5g, Carbs: 5g, Fats: 31g

29.   Warm Strawberry Coconut Flakes

Ingredients:

¼ cup of flaked coconut, lightly toasted

1 cup of almond milk (you can use coconut almond milk for some extra flavor)

1 tbsp of chia seeds

1 tbsp of almonds, minced

1 tbsp of coconut oil

1 tsp of strawberry extract

½ tsp of sugar

Preparation:

Preheat the oven to 350 degrees. Line some baking paper over a baking sheet and grease with melted coconut oil.

Pour the flakes onto the sheet and toast for 10-15 minutes. Remove from the oven and transfer to a bowl.

Add almond milk, minced almonds, chia seeds, strawberry extract, and sugar. Give it a good stir and serve warm.

Nutritional information per serving: Kcal: 175 , Protein: 3.1g, Carbs: 8.6g, Fats: 19g

30.   Feta Frittata

Ingredients:

4 large red bell peppers, cut into bite-sized pieces, seeds and pulp removed

2 garlic cloves, crushed

3 large eggs

1 oz Feta cheese, crumbled

¼ cup of parsley, finely chopped

¼ cup of sour cream

¼ tsp of salt

¼ tsp of black pepper, ground

1 tbsp of extra virgin olive oil

Preparation:

Place chopped peppers in a large bowl. Season with some finely chopped parsley, salt, and pepper. Stir all well and set aside.

Preheat the oven to 370°F.

Whisk the eggs in another bowl. Add cheese, sour cream, and olive oil. Mix well with a fork. Pour the mixture over the vegetables and give it a good stir.

Grease the large baking sheet with olive oil and make a fine layer.

Bake for about 45-50 minutes. Remove from the oven and chill for at least ten minutes. Top with some sliced tomato, but this is optional.

Enjoy!

Nutritional information per serving: Kcal: 201, Protein: 29.2g, Carbs: 6.8g, Fats: 10.5g

31.   Oven-Baked Lamb Legs

Ingredients:

4 lamb legs

1 cup of spring onions, chopped

3 medium-sized potatoes, peeled and chopped

6 tbsp of olive oil

4 cups of bone broth

1 large red onion, chopped

3 garlic cloves, crushed

3 tbsp of fresh rosemary, finely chopped

2 tsp of Himalayan salt

½ tsp of black pepper, ground

½ tsp of chili pepper, ground

Preparation:

Preheat the oven to 325°F.

Place the meat in a large bowl. Add salt and pepper and gently rub into the meat.

Preheat 2 tablespoons of oil in a large nonstick frying pan and add meat. Cook for 5 minutes, stirring occasionally. Add garlic, red onions, and spring onions. Cook for 5 minutes more, or until meat golden brown. Remove from the heat.

Add the remaining oil in a large baking dish. Transfer the meat and vegetables with all its liquid to the dish. Add all other ingredients and place it in the oven. Cook for 1 hour and add water if you like it more juicier. Remove from the oven and serve warm.

Nutritional information per serving: Kcal: 252, Protein: 14.9g, Carbs: 16.9g, Fats: 14.2g

32.   Goji Smoothie

Ingredients:

1 cup of Greek yogurt

¼ cup of Goji berries

2 tbsp of chia seeds

½ tsp of cinnamon, ground

1 tsp of coconut oil

2 mint leaves, for garnish

Preparation:

Combine all ingredients in a food processor and blend until nicely smooth. Transfer to a serving glasses and garnish with mint leaves. Refrigerate for 30 minutes before serving.

Nutritional information per serving: Kcal: 472, Protein: 24.2g, Carbs: 54.7g, Fats: 19.5g

33.   Creamy Salmon Omelet

Ingredients:

6 large eggs

4 oz of salmon fillets, thinly sliced

1 cup of Cheddar cheese, crumbled

2 tbsp of olive oil

2 garlic cloves, minced

1 tbsp of fresh parsley, finely chopped

1 tbsp of fresh rosemary, finely chopped

1 tsp of Himalayan salt

½ tsp of red pepper flakes

Preparation:

In a large bowl, whisk eggs, parsley, rosemary, salt, and red pepper. Add crumbled cheese and stir once more. Set aside.

Preheat the oil in a large nonstick frying pan over a medium-high temperature. Add garlic and stir-fry for 3 minutes. Add salmon fillets and cook for 3-4 minutes on each side.

Pour the egg mixture and cook for 3-4 minutes on each side, or until eggs are set. remove from the heat and fold the omelet. Serve immediately.

Nutritional information per serving: Kcal: 433, Protein: 29.5g, Carbs: 2.9g, Fats: 34.3g

34.   Turkey with Homemade Mayonnaise

Ingredients:

1 lb of turkey breasts, thinly sliced

3 large egg yolks

1 cup of white rice, long-grained

1 tbsp of fresh parsley, finely chopped

3 tbsp of apple cider vinegar

3 tbsp of Dijon Mustard

1 cup of olive oil

1 tsp of vegetable seasoning mix

½ tsp of sea salt

Preparation:

Combine rice and 2 cups of water in a heavy-bottomed pot. Bring it to a boil and then reduce the heat to medium-low. Sprinkle with some vegetable seasoning mix and cook for 15 minutes more, or until set. Remove from the heat and set aside.

Combine egg yolks, vinegar, mustard, oil, and salt in a large bowl. Stir well to blend and set aside.

Meanwhile, melt the butter in a large frying pan over a medium-high temperature. Add meat and sprinkle with parsley and salt. Cook for 5 minutes on each side, or until golden brown. Remove from the heat and place it on a serving plate together with rice. Pour the mayonnaise over and serve.

Nutritional information per serving: Kcal: 616, Protein: 20.2g, Carbs: 34.4g, Fats: 45.2g

35.   Beef Steak Wraps

Ingredients:

1 lbs of lean beef steak

1 cup of basmati rice

2 small carrots, shredded

½ cup of spring onions, chopped

4 tbsp of olive oil

2 tbsp of balsamic vinegar

1 tsp of dried oregano, ground

½ tsp of chili pepper, ground

1 tsp of sea salt

1 head of Romaine lettuce, whole

Preparation:

Combine vinegar, 2 tablespoons of oil, oregano, chili, and salt in a large bowl. Add meat and coat well with marinade. Cover with plastic wrap and refrigerate for 2 hours.

Place the rice in a deep pot. Add about 3 cups of water and bring it to a boil. Reduce the heat to low, cover with a lid, and cook for 15 minutes, or until nicely tender. Set aside.

Now, preheat the remaining oil in a large frying pan and add the meat. Cook for 8-10 minutes on each side, or until golden brown. Remove from the heat and reserve the pan. Make thin slices and set aside.

In the same pan, carrots and spring onions. Cook for 5 minutes, stirring constantly. Remove from the heat and mix it with rice.

On a large lettuce leaf, spoon the rice mixture and top with beef steak slices. Sprinkle with extra salt and pepper to taste if needed. Wrap and secure with a toothpick. Serve immediately.

Nutritional information per serving: Kcal: 422, Protein: 30.8g, Carbs: 34.5g, Fats: 17.3g

36.   Baked Creamy Cheddar and Tomato Avocado

Ingredients:

1 ripe avocado

1 large tomato, finely chopped

1 large onion, peeled and finely chopped

2 tbsp of extra virgin olive oil

2 tbsp of tomato paste, sugar-free

¼ cup of cheddar, shredded

1 tbsp of fresh lime juice

½ tsp of salt

1 tsp of cayenne pepper

Preparation:

Preheat the oven to 350 degrees. Line some baking paper over a baking sheet and set aside.

Slice the avocado in half and remove the stone. Using a sharp knife, cut criss-cross patterns to allow the spices to penetrate the avocado flesh.

In a medium-sized skillet, heat up the olive oil over medium-high heat. Stir-fry the onion for 2-3 minutes, or until translucent, and add chopped tomato. Continue to cook until fork tender. Now add tomato paste, fresh lime juice, salt, and cayenne pepper. Give it a final stir and remove from the heat.

Fill each avocado half with this mixture and top with cheddar. Bake for 20 minutes.

Nutritional information per serving: Kcal: 252, Protein: 7.6g, Carbs: 14.1g, Fats: 19.8g

37.   Baked Zucchini with Blue Cheese Drizzle

Ingredients:

1 medium-sized zucchini, sliced lengthwise

2 large eggs

¼ cup of almond milk

½ cup of almond flour

2 garlic cloves, crushed

1 tsp of dried oregano, crushed

½ cup of gorgonzola

1 tsp of salt

½ tsp of pepper

¼ cup of extra virgin olive oil

Preparation:

Preheat the oven to 350 degrees. Grease a quarter-sized sheet pan with some olive oil and set aside.

Combine the remaining oil with crushed garlic, oregano, and pepper. Set aside.

Slice the zucchini lengthwise and sprinkle with some salt. Set aside for 5-7 minutes. Rinse well and pat dry. Arrange a single layer in a baking dish. Using a kitchen brush, spread the olive oil mixture over each zucchini slice and bake for 20 minutes.

Meanwhile, whisk together eggs, almond milk, and almond flour. Beat well with an electric mixer on high until well incorporated. Spread this mixture over zucchini and continue to cook for five more minutes.

Place gorgonzola in a microwave for two minutes. Drizzle over zucchini and serve warm.

Nutritional information per serving: Kcal: 340, Protein: 19g, Carbs: 7.3g, Fats: 35g

38.   Shiitake Casserole

Ingredients:

1lb shiitake mushrooms, whole

6 eggs

2 medium onions, peeled

3 garlic cloves, crushed

¼ cup of olive oil

½ tsp of sea salt

¼ tsp of freshly ground black pepper

Preparation:

Preheat the oven to 350 degrees. Spread 2 tbsp of olive oil over an eighth-sized baking sheet. Place the shiitake on a baking sheet. Bake for about 10-12 minutes. Remove from the oven and allow it to cool for a while. Lower the oven heat to 200 degrees.

Meanwhile, peel and finely chop the onions. Separate egg whites from yolks. Slice shiitake into ½ inch thick slices and place in a bowl. Add chopped onions, olive oil, egg whites, crushed garlic, salt, and pepper. Mix well.

Spread this mixture on a baking sheet and bake for another 15-20 minutes.

Nutritional information per serving: Kcal: 319, Protein: 41g, Carbs: 14g, Fats: 34g

39.   Pecan Quinoa Porridge

Ingredients:

2 cups of rolled oats

1 cup of white quinoa

1 cup of skim milk

1 tbsp of coconut, shredded

¼ cup of prunes, chopped

½ cup of maple syrup

1 tbsp of honey, raw

4 tbsp of pecans, roughly chopped

1 tsp of cinnamon, ground

1 tsp of vanilla extract

Preparation:

Preheat the oven to 350°F.

Combine quinoa, oats, and pecans in a large bowl.

In a separate bowl combine syrup, cinnamon, honey and vanilla extract. Now, pour this mixture into a bowl with dry ingredients and stir well to combine.

Grease a medium baking sheet with some cooking spray. Pour the previously made mixture and spread in one even layer. Bake for about 15 minutes, stirring occasionally. Remove from the oven and let it cool for a while. Transfer to a serving bowl and stir in milk and prunes. Sprinkle with shredded coconut and serve.

Nutritional information per serving: Kcal: 557, Protein: 14.8g, Carbs: 97.7g, Fats: 12.9g

40.   Lean Veal with Ginger Stew

Ingredients:

10 oz of lean veal, cut into bite-sized pieces

1 cup of tomatoes, diced

2 large potatoes, peeled and cubed

1 tbsp of fresh ginger, minced

2 tbsp of olive oil

1 small eggplant, finely chopped

1 small zucchini, finely chopped

1 small bell pepper, finely chopped

1 large onion, finely chopped

3 tbsp of tomato paste

½ cup of peanut butter

3 cups of chicken stock

1 tsp of cayenne pepper, ground

½ tsp of salt

¼ tsp of black pepper, ground

Preparation:

Preheat the oil in a large frying pan over a medium-high temperature. Add meat and cook for 4-5 minutes, or until slightly browned. Now, transfer the meat to a deep pot and set aside. In the same pan, add zucchini, tomatoes, onion, and sprinkle with ginger, salt, and pepper. Stir well and cook for 5-7 minutes. Transfer all to the pot with meat. Now, add all other ingredients. Add water to adjust thickness. Bring it to a boil and then reduce the heat to low. Cover with a lid and cook for 45-50 minutes. Remove from the heat and serve warm.

Nutritional information per serving: Kcal: 294, Protein: 16.1g, Carbs: 27.3g, Fats: 14.9g

41.   Quick Ziti with Veggies

Ingredients:

1 lb of ziti pasta

1 medium-sized cucumber, chopped

2 cups of tomatoes, diced

1 cup of sour cream

1cup of skim milk

1 tsp of dried oregano, ground

1 tbsp of olive oil

1 tbsp of balsamic vinegar

1 tsp of sea salt

¼ tsp of black pepper, ground

Preparation:

Cook pasta using package instructions. Sprinkle with some salt while cooking. Remove from the heat and drain well. Set aside.

Combine all other ingredients in a large bowl. Stir well to combine and pour over the pasta. Toss well to coat and serve immediately.

Nutritional information per serving: Kcal: 355, Protein: 12.0g, Carbs: 49.4g, Fats: 12.3g

42. Sweet Orange Asparagus

Ingredients:

1lb fresh asparagus, woody ends trimmed

2 medium onions, peeled and finely chopped

2 small jalapeno peppers, sliced

1 cup of vegetable stock

¼ cup of fresh lime juice

1 tsp of pure orange extract, sugar-free

5 tbsp of extra virgin olive oil

1 tsp of dried rosemary, crushed

Preparation:

Heat up the olive oil in a large saucepan. Add chopped onions and stir-fry for 2-3 minutes, or until translucent.

Place jalapeno peppers, lime juice, orange extract, and rosemary in a food processor. Add about ½ cup of vegetable stock and pulse until smooth. Pour the mixture into a frying pan and reduce the heat to minimum. Simmer for ten minutes.

When most of the liquid has evaporated, add trimmed asparagus and the remaining vegetable stock. Bring it to a boil and simmer until asparagus is fork tender.

Serve warm.

Nutritional information per serving: Kcal: 180, Protein: 4.9g, Carbs: 7g, Fats: 41g

43.   Greek Style Creamy Cauliflower

Ingredients:

1lb cauliflower florets

1 cup of sour cream

1 cup of Greek yogurt

1 tbsp of garlic powder

2 eggs

½ tsp of sea salt

1 tbsp of dried parsley

2 tbsp of olive oil

Preparation:

Preheat the oven to 400 degrees. Grease an eighth-sized baking sheet with some olive oil and line cauliflower florets in a single layer.

In a medium-sized bowl, combine sour cream with Greek yogurt, eggs, garlic powder, salt, and dry parsley in a bowl. Add one cup of vegetable broth and give it a good stir.

Pour over cauliflower and cook for 35 minutes, or until the liquid has evaporated and cauliflower is lightly charred and creamy.

Nutritional information per serving: Kcal: 330, Protein: 24.2g, Carbs: 15g, Fats: 43g

44.   Thai Stripped Vegetables

Ingredients:

1 pound of button mushrooms, sliced

1 medium red bell pepper, cut into strips

1 medium green bell pepper, cut into strips

7-8 cauliflower florets

½ cup of parmesan cheese

7-8 brussel sprouts, halved

1 tbsp fresh tomato sauce, sugar-free

1 fire-roasted tomato, roughly chopped

1 tsp of salt

4 tbsp of extra virgin olive oil

Preparation:

Thoroughly wash and slice mushrooms lengthwise.

In a large wok pan, heat up the olive oil over a medium-high temperature. Add cauliflower florets and brussel sprouts and cook for ten minutes, stirring constantly. Now add stripped peppers, fire-roasted tomato, salt, tomato sauce, and parmesan cheese. Give it a good stir and cook for ten more minutes.

Now you can add mushrooms and continue to cook for 5-7 more minutes. Give it a final stir and serve warm.

Nutritional information per serving: Kcal: 313, Protein: 18.9g, Carbs: 14g, Fats: 32g

45.   Hot Chili Stew

Ingredients:

2 pounds of cauliflower florets

1 tbsp chili pepper, ground

1 tablespoon of vegetable oil

6 oz tomato paste, sugar-free

2 jalapeno peppers, cut into strips

1 large tomato, roughly chopped

1 large onion, peeled and finely chopped

1 cup of fresh button mushrooms, sliced

¼ tbsp of salt

1 bay leaf

2 ½ cups vegetable broth

1 tsp of dry thyme

3 garlic cloves, crushed

Preparation:

Take a frying pan and set it over high heat. Heat up the vegetable oil and add the cauliflower florets to it. Cook, stirring constantly, until properly brown. Transfer to a deep pot. In the same pan, fry the onions, turning the heat to medium. Cook the onions for 5 minutes.

Now add jalapeno peppers, tomato paste, chili pepper, garlic, and salt. Continue to cook for 3-4 minutes. Transfer to a pot.

Add the remaining ingredients and cover with a lid. Set the heat to minimum and cook for one hour.

Nutritional information per serving: Kcal: 180, Protein: 13g, Carbs: 25g, Fats: 8.9g

46.   Turkey Rice Patties

Ingredients:

10 oz of turkey breast, finely chopped

¾ cup of chia seeds

¾ of a cup of basmati rice

¾ of a cup of buckwheat bread crumbs

1 tsp of tarragon

1 tsp of fresh parsley, finely chopped

1 tsp of garlic, minced

1 cup of fresh spinach, chopped

1 tbsp of butter

½ tsp of salt

Preparation:

Pour 1 cup of water in a small saucepan. Bring it to a boil and cook rice until it's slightly sticky. This should take about 10 minutes.

At the same time, cook chia seeds until soft in a separate pot. Finely chop the meat. Thoroughly rinse spinach.

Sprinkle with some salt and mix all the ingredients together in a large bowl. Put the bowl into the fridge to chill for 15-30 minutes.

Take mixture out of the fridge and form into patties. Make sure cooking surfaces are cleaned and greased before adding patties to prevent them from sticking.

Melt the butter in a large frying pan over a medium high temperature. Place the patties in it and fry for about 5-7 minutes on each side.

Nutritional information per serving: Kcal: 812, Protein: 38.5g, Carbs: 145.2g, Fats: 38.2g

47.   White Beans Stew

Ingredients:

2 cups of white beans, pre-cooked

2 large potatoes, peeled and chopped

1 large bell pepper, chopped

1 medium-sized tomato, diced

2 tbsp of all-purpose flour

2 tbsp of olive oil

1 small onion, chopped

1 tbsp of fresh parsley, finely chopped

1 tbsp of Cayenne pepper, ground

½ tsp of Himalayan salt

¼ tsp of black pepper, ground

Preparation:

Place the beans in a deep pot. Add enough water to cover and cook for about 2-3 minutes. Remove from the heat, drain, and rinse well. Wash the pot and pour fresh water in it. Add boiled beans and cook again for about 45 minutes, or until soften.

Preheat the oil in a heavy-bottomed pot over a medium-high temperature. Add the onion and stir-fry until translucent. Add beans, potatoes, tomato, bell pepper, parsley, chili, salt, and pepper. Add enough water to cover all ingredients. Bring it to a boil then reduce the heat to low. Cover with a lid and cook for 1 hour.

In a small saucepan, combine cayenne pepper, flour and about 3 tablespoons of water. Stir well and bring it to a boil. Remove from the heat and stir into the pot. Cook for 10 more minutes and remove from the heat. Serve warm.

Nutritional information per serving: Kcal: 376, Protein: 18.7g, Carbs: 65.9g, Fats: 5.6g

48.   English Spinach Pie

Ingredients:

1 pack (9 oz) of fresh spinach, chopped

7oz dandelion leaves, torn

4 whole eggs

½ cup of coconut milk

2 oz of crumbled Feta cheese

¼ cup grated Parmesan cheese

½ cup shredded Mozzarella cheese

3 tbsp of vegetable oil

1 tsp of salt

½ tsp of black pepper

Preparation:

Preheat the oven to 350°F. Lightly grease a baking dish with vegetable oil and set aside.

Whisk the eggs thoroughly in a mixing bowl. Gradually whisk in the milk and beat well on high. Add parmesan and continue to beat until well combined. Set aside.

Place the chopped spinach and dandelion in the greased baking dish and add crumbled Feta cheese. Pour in the egg mixture and cover the other ingredients completely.

Bake for about 40 to 45 minutes or until the cheese has melted and lightly browned.

Remove from the oven and chill for 10-15 minutes before serving.

Nutritional information per serving: Kcal: 190, Protein: 15g, Carbs: 8g, Fats: 20g

49.   Balsamic Mushrooms

Ingredients:

1 lb of button mushrooms, halved

3 tbsp of extra-virgin olive oil

1 tbsp of stevia, powdered

1 tbsp of Dijon mustard

1 tbsp of balsamic vinegar

1 tsp of lemon juice

1 tbsp of fresh rosemary, finely chopped

¼ tsp of salt

¼ tsp of black pepper, ground

Preparation:

Combine oil, stevia, vinegar, mustard, salt, and pepper in a large bowl. Stir well and add mushrooms. Coat well the mushrooms and set aside for 30 minutes to allow flavors to meld.

Preheat the electric grill over a medium-high temperature. Transfer mushrooms to the grill and reserve the marinade.

Grill mushrooms for 5 minutes, stirring constantly and transfer to a serving plate. Drizzle with marinade leftovers and serve with some steamed vegetables.

Nutritional information per serving: Kcal: 240, Protein: 7.3g, Carbs: 5.8g, Fats: 28g

50.   Stuffed Mozzarella Tomatoes

Ingredients:

4 large tomatoes, whole

1 cup of Mozzarella cheese, crumbled

½ cup of onion, finely chopped

10 of spinach, finely chopped

2 tbsp of Parmesan cheese, grated

1tbsp of fresh parsley, finely chopped

2 tbsp of olive oil

½ tsp of salt

¼ tsp of black pepper, ground

Preparation:

Preheat the oven to 400°F.

Carefully place spinach in a pot of boiling water. Cook for 1 minute and remove from the heat. Drain well set aside.

Hollow out the tomatoes and reserve the pulp. Remove the seeds out of the pulp and chop it into a large mixing bowl. Stir in the spinach, Mozzarella, Parmesan, salt, and pepper.

Spoon the mixture into the tomatoes and place them into a previously greased baking dish. Bake for 5 minutes and remove from the heat.

Enjoy!

Nutrition information per serving: Kcal: 159, Protein: 14.5g, Carbs: 12.9g, Fats: 10.8g

51.   Shiitake Scallopini with Gorgonzola Sauce

Ingredients:

1lb shiitake mushrooms

¼ cup of butter

1 garlic clove, crushed

1 tsp of dry oregano

¼ cup of fresh lime juice

1 cup of button mushrooms, sliced

½ cup of Gorgonzola cheese, chopped

½ cup of sour cream

3 tbsp of Parmesan cheese, grated

½ tsp of salt

½ cup of all-purpose flour

Preparation:

In a small bowl, combine the almond flour with sour cream, butter, parmesan cheese, and gorgonzola. Add fresh lime juice and beat well with electric mixer, on high.

Season shiitake with salt and oregano. Place in a heavy bottomed saucepan. Add the creamy mixture, button mushrooms, and garlic.

Cover and cook for 30 minutes over medium-low heat.

Nutritional information per serving: Kcal: 300, Protein: 24.5g, Carbs: 12g, Fats: 36g

52. Italian Garlic Cauliflower Pasta

Ingredients:

6 cups of cauliflower florets

3 large ripe tomatoes

3 tbsp of extra virgin olive oil

2 garlic cloves, crushed

½ tsp of dry oregano

¼ tsp of salt

¼ cup of fresh lime juice

½ cup of all-purpose flour

1 cup of vegetable broth

Preparation:

Preheat the oven to 350 degrees.

Place cauliflower in a deep pot and add enough water to cover. Boil until dente. Remove from the heat and drain. Set aside.

Whisk together vegetable broth with flour. Set aside.

Peel and roughly chop the tomatoes. Make sure you keep all the liquid.

Heat up the olive oil over a medium temperature. Add the garlic and stir-fry for several minutes. Now add tomatoes, oregano, and salt. Reduce the heat to low and cook until the tomatoes have softened. Add lime juice and cook for 10 more minutes stirring constantly. Turn off the heat, add cauliflower and cover.

Let it stand for 10 minutes and transfer to a lightly greased baking sheet. Evenly pour over the vegetable broth.

Bake for 15-20 minutes or until you get a nice color on top.

Nutritional information per serving: Kcal: 93, Protein: 5g, Carbs: 15g, Fats: 14g

53.   Goat's Cheese Salad

Ingredients:

5 cherry tomatoes, whole

A handful of black olives

1 medium-sized onion, peeled and sliced

3.5 oz fresh goat's cheese

2 radishes, sliced

3.5 oz of lamb's lettuce

2 tbsp of freshly squeezed lime juice

3 tbsp of extra virgin olive oil

Salt to taste

Preparation:

Place the vegetables in a large bowl. Add olive oil, goat's cheese, fresh lime juice and some salt to taste. Toss to combine.

Nutritional information per serving: Kcal: 225, Protein: 18.5g, Carbs: 10g, Fats: 35g

54.   Cottage Cheese Fried Zucchini

Ingredients:

2 small zucchinis, sliced lengthwise

½ cup of cottage cheese

1 cup of lamb's lettuce

1 cup of cherry tomatoes

½ cup of button mushrooms, sliced

1 tsp of salt

½ tsp of freshly ground black pepper

2 tbsp of olive oil

Preparation:

Wash and pat dry the zucchini with some kitchen paper. Slice lengthwise.

Use a large grill pan and grease it with some olive oil. Heat up over medium-high heat and sliced zucchinis. Grill for 3-4 minutes on each side, remove from the heat and chill for a while.

Meanwhile, add mushrooms into the grill pan and grill until the liquid evaporates. Remove from the heat and chill for a while.

Place lamb's lettuce, cottage cheese, and cherry tomatoes in a large bowl. Add grilled zucchini, mushrooms, and season with salt and pepper. Toss to combine and serve.

Nutritional information per serving: Kcal: 220, Protein: 27g, Carbs: 14g, Fats: 24g

55.   Warm Broccoli Slaw

Ingredients:

12 oz bag broccoli slaw

½ cup of brussel sprouts, halved

½ cup of cauliflower, chopped

A handful of finely chopped kale

3 tbsp of sesame oil

1 tsp of ginger, grated

½ tsp of salt

¼ cup of goat milk yogurt

Preparation:

Heat up the oil in a large skillet. Add brussel sprouts and chopped cauliflower. Cook for 10-15 minutes, stirring constantly.

Stir in broccoli slaw, grated ginger, salt, and kale. Add about ¼ cup of water and continue to cook for another 10 minutes. When the water has evaporated, stir in yogurt and remove from the heat.

Serve warm.

Nutritional information per serving: Kcal: 214, Protein: 9g, Carbs: 13g, Fats: 15g

56.   Warm Vegetable Kebab

Ingredients:

1 lb cauliflower florets, halved

2 large onions, grated

5 tbsp of extra virgin olive oil

½ tsp of red pepper, crushed

½ tsp of dried oregano

¼ tsp of salt

¼ tsp of ground black pepper

1 tbsp of tomato sauce

2 cups of lukewarm water

1 large tomato, sliced into wedges

½ green pepper, chopped

1 cup of plain yogurt, or sour cream

Preparation:

First, put the onions into a blender and blend until smooth. Transfer the liquid from the blender into a large bowl, and remove the remaining pulp.

Cut the cauliflower florets and slice it into bite-sized pieces.

Combine the spices with two tablespoons of olive oil and onions. Stir well. Now add the cauliflower and stir all together. Cover the lid and set aside.

Now, preheat the remaining olive oil over a medium temperature. Add the tomato sauce and stir well. If you're a fan of spicy food, you can add a pinch of crushed chili pepper. This, however, is optional. Now add the water, a pinch of salt, and gently simmer for a couple of minutes. Remove from the heat and set aside.

Meanwhile, heat up 2 tablespoons of vegetable oil and add the cauliflower. Stir-fry for about ten minutes. Now add the tomato sauce and onions. Stir well and cook for another five minutes. Set aside.

Place the cauliflower pieces onto a serving platter, top with tomato and pepper, and serve with some yogurt or sour cream.

Enjoy!

Nutritional information per serving: Kcal: 190, Protein: 12g, Carbs: 21g, Fats: 22g

57.   Tomato Cumin Soup

Ingredients:

1 pound of fresh tomatoes, peeled and finely chopped

3 large cucumbers, finely chopped

3 spring onions, finely chopped

1 medium-sized red onion, finely chopped

1 tbsp of tomato paste, sugar-free

½ tsp of salt

1 tbsp of ground cumin

¼ tsp of pepper

Fresh parsley, for serving

Preparation:

Preheat the non-stick frying pan over a medium-high temperature. Add the onions and stir-fry for 3-4 minutes. Now add the tomatoes, tomato paste, cucumber, cumin, salt, and pepper. Cook for another five minutes, or until caramelized.

Add three cups of lukewarm water, reduce the heat to minimum and cook for about 15 minutes. Now add about

1 cup of water and bring it to a boil. Remove from the heat and serve with fresh parsley.

Serve cold.

Nutritional information per serving: Kcal: 160, Protein: 6g, Carbs: 27g, Fats: 0.9g

58.   Sweet Almond Patties

Ingredients:

1lb cauliflower florets, sliced

7oz almonds, toasted

1 cup of almond milk

1 egg

1 tsp of sea salt

1 tbsp of almond butter

1 cup of almond flour

½ cup of parsley, finely chopped

½ cup of plain yogurt

olive oil

Preparation:

Place cauliflower florets in a deep pot. Add enough water to cover and bring it to a boil. Cook until fork tender. Remove from the heat and transfer to a bowl. Add one teaspoon of salt, almond milk, and almond butter. Mash until a smooth puree. Set aside.

Finely chop the almonds and combine with cauliflower puree. Add almond flour, eggs, and parsley. Mix until well combined. Using your hands, shape 1-inch thick patties.

Preheat some oil over a medium-high heat. Fry each patty for about 2-3 minutes on each side.

Nutritional information per serving: Kcal: 322, Protein: 17g, Carbs: 18g, Fats: 28g

59.   Spring Greens

Ingredients:

3.5oz fresh chicory, torn

3.5oz wild asparagus, finely chopped

3.5oz Swiss chard, torn

A handful of fresh mint, chopped

A handful of rocket salad, torn

3 garlic cloves, crushed

¼ tsp of freshly ground black pepper

1 tsp of salt

¼ cup of fresh lemon juice

Olive oil

Preparation:

Fill a large pot with salted water and add greens. Bring it to a boil and cook for 2-3 minutes. Remove from the heat and drain.

In a medium-sized skillet, heat up 3 tablespoons of olive oil. Add crushed garlic and stir-fry for about 2-3 minutes. Now add the greens, salt, pepper, and about half of the lemon juice. Stir-fry the greens for five more minutes.

Remove from the heat. Season with more lemon juice and serve.

Nutritional information per serving: Kcal: 55, Protein: 4g, Carbs: 7g, Fats: 8g

60. Creamy Coconut Manicotti

Ingredients:

5 crepes

¼ cup of coconut oil

3oz coconut flour

2pts coconut milk

8.8oz ricotta cheese

3oz grated Parmesan cheese

5oz fresh spinach, torn

Seasoning to taste

Preparation:

Preheat the oven to 350 degrees.

Bring the coconut oil, flour and milk slowly to a boil, whisking constantly until thickened. Put half of the sauce into a bowl and mix with ricotta, parmesan, spinach, and seasoning to taste.

Lay a crepe on the work surface. Spoon out about 1/5 of the mixture and place it on a crepe. Roll up the crepe and place it on a baking sheet. Repeat the process until you have used all the ingredients.

Bake for 10 minutes, remove from the oven and serve.

Nutritional information per serving: Kcal: 500, Protein: 31g, Carbs: 11.5g, Fats: 50g

61.   Garlic Grilled Zucchini

Ingredients:

1 large zucchini

3 eggs

1 tsp of dried rosemary

2 garlic cloves, crushed

¼ tsp of sea salt

1 tbsp of olive oil

Preparation:

Peel zucchini and cut into 1 inch thick slices. Sprinkle some salt set aside for 15 minutes. Rinse well and pat dry using a kitchen paper.

In a large bowl, whisk together eggs with crushed garlic and rosemary.

Heat up the olive oil in frying pan over a medium temperature.

Soak the zucchini slices in the egg mixture. Make few holes with a knife to allow the mixture to permeate the eggplant.

Fry it until golden brown color, on each side. This should take about 10 minutes. Serve your zucchini warm.

Nutritional information per serving: Kcal: 198, Protein: 13g, Carbs: 7g, Fats: 25g

121 Complete Weight Gaining Shake and Meal Recipes to Get Bigger and Stronger

62.   Tomato Soup with Fresh Basil

Ingredients:

2oz tomato, peeled and roughly chopped

Ground black pepper to taste

1 tbsp of celery, finely chopped

1 onion, diced

1 tbsp of fresh basil, finely chopped

Fresh water

Preparation:

Preheat the non-stick frying pan over a medium-high temperature. Add the onions, celery, and fresh basil. Sprinkle some pepper and stir-fry for about 10 minutes, until caramelized.

Add the tomato and about ¼ cup of water. Reduce the heat to minimum and cook for about 15 minutes, until softened. Now add about 1 cup of water and bring it to a boil. Remove from the heat and serve with fresh parsley.

Nutrition information per serving: Kcal: 25, Protein: 0.7g, Carbs: 4.9g, Fats: 0.9g

121

63.   Cocoa Butter Protein Bars

Ingredients:

1 cup of toasted almonds, finely chopped

½ cup of cocoa butter

½ cup of sugar

2 tablespoons of chia seeds

¼ cup of raw cocoa powder

3 egg whites

¼ cup of coconut milk

Preparation:

Combine the ingredients in a bowl and mix well to combine. Shape the balls using your hands and refrigerate for about 30 minutes.

Nutritional information per serving: Kcal: 260, Protein: 11g, Carbs: 9g, Fats: 28g

64.   Salad 'Del Chef'

Ingredients:

3 large eggs

½ cucumber, sliced

1 small tomato, roughly chopped

1 cup of fresh lettuce, torn

1 small green pepper, sliced

½ tsp salt

1 tbsp of lime juice

3 tbsp of olive oil

Preparation:

Hard boil the eggs for 10 minutes. Remove from the heat, rinse and chill for a while. Gently peel and slice each egg. Transfer to a large jar.

Now, combine the vegetables in a glass jar. Add the meat and mix well. Season with salt and some lime juice. Seal the lid and you're ready to go.

Nutritional information per serving: Kcal: 55, Protein: 7g, Carbs: 2.8g, Fats: 11.3g

65.   Ginger Chia Smoothie

Ingredients:

1 cup of milk

1 tbsp of coconut oil

1 tbsp of chia seeds

1 tsp of ginger, ground

2 tsp of sugar

1 tsp of pure peach extract

Preparation:

Combine the ingredients in a blender and pulse to combine. You can add some ice cubes, but this is optional. Serve cold.

Nutritional information per serving: Kcal: 417, Protein: 6g, Carbs: 10g, Fats: 41g

66.　Super Healthy Beet Greens Salad

Ingredients:

8 oz leek, chopped into bite-size pieces

A handful of beet greens

1 large tomato, chopped

2 garlic cloves, finely chopped

3 tbsp of vegetable oil

A few mint leaves

½ tsp of salt

½ tsp of red pepper

½ tsp of Cayenne pepper

Preparation:

Heat up some vegetable oil in a large skillet. Stir-fry the garlic for 2-3 minutes, or until lightly charred. Now add leek, salt, pepper, and cayenne pepper. Cook for ten minutes, over medium heat, stirring constantly. Remove from the heat and transfer to a bowl.

Add a handful of beet greens, chopped tomato, and fresh mint. Toss well to combine and serve.

Nutritional information per serving: Kcal: 133, Protein: 2.1g, Carbs: 15g, Fats: 15.5g

67.   Coconut Detox Smoothie

Ingredients:

1 cup of coconut water

¼ cup of baby spinach, finely chopped

¼ cup of green tea

¼ cup of small – sized cucumber, peeled and chopped

¼ medium-sized avocado, chopped

1 tsp organic vanilla extract

2 tsp of sugar

Preparation:

Combine the ingredients in a blender for about 40 seconds and chill well before serving.

Nutritional information per serving: Kcal: 110, Protein: 4.2g, Carbs: 8.5g, Fats: 3.4g

68.   Coconut Yogurt with Chia Seeds and Almonds

Ingredients:

1 cup of coconut yogurt

3 tbsp of chia seeds

1 tsp of toasted almonds, finely chopped

2 tsp of honey

Preparation:

For this easy recipe, combine 3 tbsp of chia seeds with 1 cup of soy yogurt, 1 tsp of ground almonds and 1 tbsp of honey. Use a fork or an electric mixer to get a smooth mixture. Allow it to cool in the refrigerator.

You can combine ¾ cup of soy yogurt with ¼ cup of rice yogurt for extra flavor.

Nutritional information per serving: Kcal: 312, Protein: 14g, Carbs: 44g, Fats: 41g

69.   Grilled Pepper Broccoli

Ingredients:

4oz fresh broccoli

Freshly ground black pepper to taste

Fresh parsley, chopped

3 tbsp of olive oil

Preparation:

Heat up the olive oil in a large grill pan. Place the broccoli and grill for 15 minutes, or until lightly charred.

Transfer to a plate and sprinkle with some pepper and parsley. Serve warm.

Serving tip:

Combine the chopped parsley with one garlic clove.

Nutritional information per serving: Kcal: 289, Protein: 3g, Carbs: 7g, Fats: 31g

JUICES

1. Celery Apple Juice

Ingredients:

1 large green apple, cored

1 large lemon, peeled

3 large celery stalks, chopped

1 large cucumber

2 oz of coconut water

Preparation:

Wash the apple and cut lengthwise in half. Remove the core and cut into small chunks. Set aside.

Peel the lemon and cut lengthwise in half. Set aside.

Wash the celery stalks and cut into small pieces. Set aside.

Peel the cucumber and cut into small chunks. Set aside.

Now, combine apple, lemon, celery, and cucumber in a juicer and process until well juiced. Transfer to serving glasses and stir in the coconut water.

Add few ice cubes and serve immediately.

Enjoy!

Nutritional information per serving: Kcal: 175, Protein: 5.1g, Carbs: 50.2g, Fats: 1.3g

2.   Mixed Berry Juice

Ingredients:

1 cup of blackberries

1 cup of blueberries

3 large strawberries, chopped

1 large lime, peeled

1 large cucumber, chopped

1 cup of fresh mint, torn

2 oz of water

Preparation:

Combine blackberries and blueberries in a colander. Rinse under cold running water and drain. Set aside.

Wash the strawberries and remove the stems, if any. Cut into bite-sized pieces and set aside.

Peel the lime and cut lengthwise in half. Set aside.

Wash the cucumber and cut into small chunks. Set aside.

Wash the mint and torn with hands. Set aside.

Now, combine blackberries, blueberries, strawberries, cucumber, and mint in a juicer and process until juiced. Transfer to serving glasses and stir in the water.

Add some ice or refrigerate for 15 minutes before serving.

Nutritional information per serving: Kcal: 173, Protein: 6.6g, Carbs: 57.8g, Fats: 1.9g

3.   Cherry Banana Juice

Ingredients:

2 cups of cherries, pitted

1 large banana, chunked

1 large lime, peeled

2 large green apples, chopped

¼ tsp of cinnamon

1 oz of water

Preparation:

Rinse the cherries under cold running water and drain. Cut each in half and remove the pits. Set aside.

Peel the banana and chop into chunks. Set aside.

Peel the lime and cut lengthwise in half. Set aside.

Wash the apples and cut lengthwise in half. Remove the core and cut into small chunks.

Now, combine cherries, banana, lime, and apples in a juicer and process until well juiced.

Transfer to a serving glass and stir in the cinnamon and water. Add some ice before serving and enjoy!

Nutritional information per serving: Kcal: 297, Protein: 4.2g, Carbs: 87.5g, Fats: 1.2g

4.   Raspberry Carrot Juice

Ingredients:

1 cup of raspberries

2 large carrots, peeled and chopped

1 large orange, wedged

¼ tsp of ginger, ground

1 tbsp of liquid honey

Preparation:

Using a colander, rinse the raspberries under cold running water and drain. Set aside.

Wash the carrots and peel them. Cut into small chunks and set aside.

Peel the orange and divide into wedges. Set aside.

Now, combine raspberries, carrots, and orange in a juicer and process until well juiced. Transfer to a serving glass and stir in the ginger and honey.

Refrigerate for 15 minutes before serving.

Nutritional information per serving: Kcal: 204, Protein: 4.5g, Carbs: 67.1g, Fats: 1.3g

5.   Apricot Orange Juice

Ingredients:

2 whole apricots, pitted

1 large orange, wedged

1 cup of green grapes

1 small ginger slice, peeled

1 oz of water

Preparation:

Wash the apricots and cut lengthwise in half. Remove the pits and cut into bite-sized pieces. Set aside.

Peel the orange and divide into wedges. Set aside.

Wash the grapes and set aside.

Peel the ginger slice and cut into small pieces. Set aside.

Now, combine apricots, orange, grapes, and ginger in a juicer. Process until juiced and transfer to a serving glass. Add some ice before serving.

Nutritional information per serving: Kcal: 157, Protein: 3.3g, Carbs: 45.7g, Fats: 0.8g

6.   Cauliflower Basil Juice

Ingredients:

1 cup of cauliflower, chopped

1 cup of fresh basil, torn

1 cup of broccoli, chopped

1 cup of beet greens, torn

1 large lemon, peeled

1 medium-sized red apple, cored

Preparation:

Trim off the outer leaves of a cauliflower. Wash it and fill and cut into small pieces. Fill the measuring cup and reserve the rest in the refrigerator.

Combine basil and beet greens in a large colander. Rinse under cold running water and drain. Torn with hands and set aside.

Wash the broccoli and chop into small pieces. Set aside.

Peel the lemon and cut lengthwise in half. Set aside.

Wash the apple and cut lengthwise in half. Remove the core and cut into bite-sized pieces. Set aside.

Now, combine cauliflower, basil, broccoli, beet greens, lemon, and apple in a juicer. Process until well juiced and transfer to a serving glass.

Add few ice cubes and serve immediately.

Nutritional information per serving: Kcal: 137, Protein: 7.3g, Carbs: 42.1g, Fats: 1.3g

7.   Ginger Artichoke Juice

Ingredients:

1 medium-sized artichoke, chopped

1 small ginger slice, peeled

3 medium-sized celery stalks

2 large kiwis, peeled

1 tbsp of liquid honey

Preparation:

Trim off the outer leaves of the artichoke using a sharp paring knife. Wash it and cut into bite-sized pieces. Set aside.

Peel the ginger slice and cut into small pieces. Set aside.

Wash the celery stalks and cut into bite-sized pieces. Set aside.

Peel the kiwis and cut lengthwise in half. Set aside.

Now, combine artichoke, ginger, celery, and kiwi in a juicer. Process until well juiced and transfer to a serving glass. Stir in the honey and refrigerate for 15 minutes before serving.

Nutritional information per serving: Kcal: 174, Protein: 6.6g, Carbs: 54.6g, Fats: 1.2g

8.   Guava Mango Juice

Ingredients:

1 large guava, chopped

1 cup of mango, chunked

1 medium-sized banana, chopped

1 large orange, wedged

1 oz of coconut water

Preparation:

Wash and peel the guava and mango. Cut into small chunks and set aside.

Peel the banana and cut into small chunks. Set aside.

Peel the orange and divide into wedges. Set aside.

Now, combine guava, mango, banana, and orange in a juicer and process until well juiced. Transfer to a serving glass and stir in the water.

Add some ice and serve immediately.

Enjoy!

Nutritional information per serving: Kcal: 275, Protein: 5.7g, Carbs: 81.1g, Fats: 1.8g

9.   Avocado Mango Juice

Ingredients:

1 cup of avocado, cubed

1 medium-sized mango

1large orange, wedged

¼ tsp of ginger, ground

3 tbsp of coconut water

Preparation:

Peel the avocado and cut lengthwise in half. Remove the pit and cut into small cubes. Fill the measuring cup and reserve the rest to a refrigerator.

Peel the mango and cut into small chunks. Set aside.

Peel the orange and divide into wedges. Cut each wedge in half and set aside.

Now, combine avocado, mango, and orange in a juicer and process until well juiced. Transfer to a serving glass and stir in the ginger and coconut water.

Add some ice and serve immediately.

Nutritional information per serving: Kcal: 457, Protein: 8.1g, Carbs: 84.7g, Fats: 23.5g

10.   Apple Carrot Juice

Ingredients:

1 medium-sized apple, cored

1 medium-sized carrot, chopped

1 whole lemon, peeled

1 large peach, pitted

2 oz of water

¼ tsp of cinnamon, ground

Preparation:

Wash the apple and cut lengthwise in half. Remove the core and cut into bite-sized pieces. Set aside.

Wash and peel the carrot. Cut into small chunks and set aside.

Peel the lemon and cut lengthwise in half. Set aside.

Wash the peach and cut in half. Remove the pit and cut into bite-sized pieces. Set aside.

Now, combine apple, carrot, lemon, and peach in a juicer. Process until nicely juiced. Transfer to a serving glass and stir in the water and cinnamon.

Add some ice or refrigerate for 10 minutes before serving.

Enjoy!

Nutritional information per serving: Kcal: 165, Protein: 3.6g, Carbs: 50.7g, Fats: 1.1g

11.   Beet Lemon Juice

Ingredients:

2 large beets, trimmed and chopped

1 whole lemon, peeled

1 cup of broccoli, chopped

1 large cucumber, sliced

Preparation:

Wash the beets and trim off the green parts. Cut into bite-sized pieces and set aside.

Peel the lemon and cut lengthwise in half. Set aside.

Wash the broccoli and cut into bite-sized pieces. Fill the measuring cup and reserve the rest for later.

Wash the cucumber and cut into thin slices. Set aside.

Now, combine beets, lemon, broccoli, and cucumber in a juicer and process until juiced. Transfer to a serving glass and add some ice before serving.

Enjoy!

Nutritional information per serving: Kcal: 123, Protein: 7.8g, Carbs: 38.1g, Fats: 1.1g

12.   Fennel Collard Green Juice

Ingredients:

1 cup of fennel, chopped

1 cup of collard greens, torn

1 large leek, chopped

1 cup of fresh mint, torn

1 large green apple, cored

A handful of spinach

1 tbsp of liquid honey

Preparation:

Wash the fennel bulb and trim off the wilted outer layers. Cut into small chunks and fill the measuring cup. Reserve the rest in the refrigerator.

In a large colander, combine collard greens, mint, and spinach. Rinse thoroughly under cold running water and drain. Torn with hands and set aside.

Wash the leek and cut into bite-sized pieces. Set aside.

Wash the apple and cut in half. Remove the core and cut into bite-sized pieces. Set aside.

Now, combine fennel, collard greens, mint, spinach, leek, and apple in a juicer. Process until well juiced.

Transfer to a serving glass and refrigerate for 15 minutes before serving.

Nutritional information per serving: Kcal: 180, Protein: 6.2g, Carbs: 53.7g, Fats: 1.4g

13.   Blueberry Banana Juice

Ingredients:

1 cup of blueberries

1 medium-sized banana, chopped

1 whole lime, peeled

1 large pear, chopped

1 cup of blackberries

1 large orange, wedged

Preparation:

In a large colander, combine blueberries and blackberries. Rinse well under cold running water and drain. Set aside.

Peel the banana and chop into chunks. Set aside.

Peel the lime and cut lengthwise in half. Set aside.

Wash the pear and cut in half. Remove the core and cut into bite-sized pieces. Set aside.

Peel the orange and divide into wedges. Set aside.

Now, combine blueberries, blackberries, banana, lime, pear, and orange in a juicer and process until well juiced.

Transfer to a serving glass and add some crushed ice.

Enjoy!

Nutritional information per serving: Kcal: 376, Protein: 7.2g, Carbs: 122.6g, Fats: 2.6g

14.   Pineapple Orange Juice

Ingredients:

1 cup of pineapple chunks

1 medium-sized orange, peeled

1 small carrot, chopped

1 whole lime, peeled

1 tbsp of liquid honey

Preparation:

Cut the top of a pineapple and peel it using a sharp knife. Cut into small chunks. Reserve the rest of the pineapple in a refrigerator.

Peel the orange and divide into wedges. Cut each wedge in half and set aside.

Peel the carrot and cut into thin slices. Set aside.

Peel the lime and cut lengthwise in half. Set aside.

Now, combine pineapple, orange, carrot, and lime in a juicer and process until well juiced. Transfer to a serving glass and stir in the honey.

Refrigerate for 15 minutes before serving.

Nutritional information per serving: Kcal: 207, Protein: 2.7g, Carbs: 61.5g, Fats: 0.7g

15. Peach Plum Juice

Ingredients:

2 medium-sized peaches, pitted

2 whole plums, pitted

1 whole lemon, peeled

1 cup of watermelon

¼ tsp of ginger, ground

Preparation:

Wash the peaches and cut in half. Remove the pits and cut into bite-sized pieces. Set aside.

Wash the plums and cut lengthwise in half. Remove the pits and set aside.

Peel the lemons and cut lengthwise in half. Set aside.

Cut the watermelon lengthwise. For one cup, you will need a large slice. Peel and cut into chunks. Remove the seeds and set aside. Reserve the rest for some other juices.

Now, combine peaches, plums, lemon, and watermelon in a juicer and process until juiced. Transfer to a serving glass and stir in the ginger.

Refrigerate for 10 minutes before serving.

Nutritional information per serving: Kcal: 205, Protein: 5.2g, Carbs: 60.6g, Fats: 1.5g

16.   Red Pepper Tomato Juice

Ingredients:

2 large red bell peppers, chopped

3 cherry tomatoes, halved

1 cup of fresh parsley, chopped

1 medium-sized carrot, sliced

1 tsp of fresh rosemary, finely chopped

Preparation:

Wash the bell peppers and cut lengthwise in half. Remove the seeds and cut into small pieces. Set aside.

Wash the tomatoes and cut in half. Set aside.

Rinse the parsley under cold running water and chop into small pieces.

Wash and peel the carrot. Cut into thin slices and set aside.

Now, combine bell peppers, tomatoes, parsley, carrot, and rosemary in a juicer and process until juiced.

Transfer to a serving glass and refrigerate for 10 minutes before serving.

Nutritional information per serving: Kcal: 112, Protein: 6.1g, Carbs: 31.4g, Fats: 1.7g

17.   Squash Kiwi Juice

Ingredients:

1 cup of crookneck squash

1 whole kiwi, peeled

1 medium-sized orange, peeled

1 cup of fresh kale, torn

1 tbsp of liquid honey

1 oz of water

Preparation:

Peel the crookneck squash and scrape out the seeds with a spoon. Cut into small cubes and fill the measuring cup. Reserve the rest of the squash for some other recipe. Wrap in a plastic foil and refrigerate.

Peel the kiwi and cut lengthwise in half. Set aside.

Peel the orange and divide into wedges. Set aside.

Rinse the kale under cold running water and slightly drain. Torn with hands and set aside.

Now, combine crookneck squash, kiwi, orange, and kale in a juicer. Process until well juiced and transfer to a serving glass.

Stir in the honey and water. Add some ice before serving and enjoy!

Nutritional information per serving: Kcal: 126, Protein: 6.2g, Carbs: 36.3g, Fats: 1.5g

18.   Asparagus Avocado Juice

Ingredients:

1 cup of fresh asparagus, trimmed

1 cup of avocado, cubed

1 whole lime, peeled

1 cup of Swiss chard, torn

1 small Golden Delicious apple, cored

1 small ginger knob, peeled

Preparation:

Wash the asparagus and trim off the woody ends. Cut into bite-sized pieces and set aside.

Peel the avocado and cut lengthwise in half. Remove the pit and cut into small chunks. Set aside.

Peel the lime and cut lengthwise in half. Set aside.

Rinse the Swiss chard thoroughly under cold running water and slightly drain. Torn with hands and set aside.

Peel the ginger knob and cut into small pieces. Set aside.

Now, process asparagus, avocado, lime, chard, and ginger in a juicer. Transfer to a serving glass and refrigerate for 15 minutes before serving.

Enjoy!

Nutritional information per serving: Kcal: 298, Protein: 7.3g, Carbs: 41.6g, Fats: 22.5g

19.   Artichoke Tomato Juice

Ingredients:

1 medium-sized artichoke, chopped

1 medium-sized tomato, chopped

1 medium-sized bell pepper, chopped

1 garlic clove, peeled

1 cup of cucumber, sliced

1 tsp of balsamic vinegar

¼ tsp of salt

Preparation:

Using a sharp knife, trim off the outer leaves of the artichoke. Wash it and cut into bite-sized pieces. Set aside.

Wash the tomato and place it in a small bowl. Cut into small pieces, but make sure to keep the juices while cutting. Set aside.

Wash the pepper and cut in half. Remove the seeds and chop into small pieces. Set aside.

Wash the cucumber and cut into thin slices. Fill the measuring cup and refrigerate the rest for later.

Now, combine artichoke, tomato, bell pepper, garlic, and cucumber in a juicer and process until juiced.

Transfer to a serving glass and stir in the vinegar and salt. You can sprinkle with some fresh rosemary for some extra taste. However, it is optional.

Refrigerate for 10 minutes before serving.

Nutritional information per serving: Kcal: 86, Protein: 7g, Carbs: 28.3g, Fats: 0.9g

20.   Brussels Sprouts Juice

Ingredients:

2 cups of Brussels sprouts, halved

1 medium-sized Granny Smith's apple, cored

1 cup of fresh mint, torn

1 cup of fresh kale, torn

1 whole lime, peeled

1 oz of water

Preparation:

Wash the Brussels sprouts and trim off the outer leaves. Cut in half and fill the measuring cup. Reserve the rest for later.

Wash the apple and cut in half. Remove the core and cut into bite-sized pieces. Set aside.

Combine mint and kale in a large colander and rinse under cold running water. Slightly drain and torn with hands. Set aside.

Peel the lime and cut lengthwise in half. Set aside.

Now, combine Brussels sprouts, apple, mint, kale, and lime in a juicer and process until juiced. Transfer to a serving glass and stir in the water.

Refrigerate for 10 minutes before serving.

Enjoy!

Nutritional information per serving: Kcal: 171, Protein: 10.6g, Carbs: 51.7g, Fats: 1.7g

21.   Parsnip Carrot Juice

Ingredients:

2 cups of parsnip, sliced

1 medium-sized carrot, sliced

1 cup of cucumber, sliced

1 cup of watercress, torn

1 whole lemon, peeled

1 small ginger knob, peeled

Preparation:

Wash and peel the parsnip and carrot. Cut into thin slices and set aside.

Peel the cucumber and chop into chunks. Fill the measuring cup and reserve the rest for later.

Rinse the watercress under cold running water and slightly drain. Torn with hands and set aside.

Peel the lemon and cut lengthwise in half. Set aside.

Peel the ginger knob and cut into small pieces. Set aside.

Now, combine parsnip, carrot, cucumber, watercress, lemon, and ginger in a juicer and process until well juiced.

Transfer to a serving glass and add few ice cubes before serving.

Nutritional information per serving: Kcal: 192, Protein: 5.6g, Carbs: 62.5g, Fats: 1.3g

22.　Cauliflower Broccoli Juice

Ingredients:

1 cup of cauliflower, chopped

1 cup of broccoli, chopped

1 small green apple, cored

1 cup of fresh kale, torn

¼ teaspoon of ginger, ground

Preparation:

Wash the cauliflower and trim off the outer leaves. Cut into small pieces and set aside.

Wash the broccoli thoroughly and chop into small pieces. Set aside.

Wash the apple and cut lengthwise in half. remove the core and cut into bite-sized pieces. Set aside.

Rinse the kale under cold running water and slightly drain. Torn with hands and set aside.

Now, combine cauliflower, broccoli, apple, and kale in a juicer and process until well juiced. Transfer to a serving glass and stir in the ground ginger.

Refrigerate for 20 minutes before serving.

Nutritional information per serving: Kcal: 131, Protein: 8.1g, Carbs: 36.8g, Fats: 1.5g

23.   Blackberry Lemon Juice

Ingredients:

1 cup of blackberries

1 whole lemon, peeled

1 cup of cucumber, sliced

1 cup of beets, sliced

1 oz of coconut water

Preparation:

Using a small colander, rinse the blackberries under cold running water. Slightly drain and set aside.

Peel the lemon and cut lengthwise in half. Set aside.

Wash the cucumber and cut into thin slices. Fill the measuring cup and reserve the rest in the refrigerator for some other juice.

Wash the beets and trim off the green parts. Cut into bite-sized pieces and fill the measuring cup. Reserve the rest for later.

Now, combine blackberries, lemon, cucumber, and beets in a juicer and process until juiced. Transfer to a serving glass and stir in the coconut water. Add some ice and serve immediately.

Nutritional information per serving: Kcal: 103, Protein: 5.2g, Carbs: 34.2g, Fats: 1.2g

24.   Fennel Asparagus Juice

Ingredients:

1 cup of fennel, chopped

1 cup of asparagus, trimmed and chopped

1 cup of avocado, sliced

2 medium-sized carrots

1 tbsp of liquid honey

Preparation:

Wash the fennel bulb and trim off the wilted outer layers. Cut into small chunks and fill the measuring cup. Reserve the rest for some other juice.

Wash the asparagus and trim off the woody ends. Cut into bite-sized pieces and fill the measuring cup. Refrigerate the rest for later.

Peel the avocado and cut lengthwise in half. Remove the pit and cut into thin slices. Fill the measuring cup and reserve the rest for later.

Wash and peel the carrots. Cut into small chunks and set aside.

Now, combine fennel, asparagus, avocado, and carrots in a juicer and process until well juiced. Transfer to a serving glass and stir in the honey.

Refrigerate for 15 minutes before serving.

Nutritional information per serving: Kcal: 263, Protein: 8.1g, Carbs: 35.7g, Fats: 22.1g

25. Cantaloupe Mango Juice

Ingredients:

1 cup of cantaloupe, diced

1 cup of mango, chunked

1 medium-sized peach, pitted

1 whole lime, peeled

1 cup of fresh mint, finely chopped

Preparation:

Cut the cantaloupe in half. Scoop out the seeds and cut two wedges and peel them. Chop into chunks and set aside. Reserve the rest of the cantaloupe in a refrigerator.

Wash and peel the mango. Cut into small chunks and set aside.

Wash the peach and cut lengthwise in half. Remove the pit and cut into bite-sized pieces. Set aside.

Peel the lime and cut lengthwise in half. Set aside.

Now, combine cantaloupe, mango, peach, lime, and mint in a juicer. Process until well juiced. Transfer to a serving glass and add some crushed ice.

Serve immediately.

Nutritional information per serving: Kcal: 205, Protein: 5.2g, Carbs: 59.2g, Fats: 1.6g

26.   Pepper Tomato Juice

Ingredients:

1 large red bell pepper, chopped

4 cherry tomatoes, halved

1 small celery stalk, chopped

1 medium-sized radish, chopped

1 small red apple, cored

¼ tsp of cayenne pepper

Preparation:

Wash the bell pepper and cut lengthwise in half. Remove the seeds and cut into small pieces. Set aside.

Wash the cherry tomatoes and place in a small bowl. Cut in half and reserve the tomato juice while cutting.

Wash the celery stalk and cut into small pieces. Set aside.

Wash the radish and trim off the green parts. Slightly peel and cut into small pieces. Set aside.

Wash the apple and cut in half. Remove the core and cut into bite-sized pieces.

Now, combine pepper, tomatoes, celery, radish, and apple in a juicer and process until well juiced. Transfer to serving glass and stir in the cayenne pepper. You can add a pinch of salt, but it's optional.

Refrigerate for 10 minutes before serving.

Nutritional information per serving: Kcal: 129, Protein: 2.9g, Carbs: 35.9g, Fats: 2.9g

27.   Avocado Cherry Juice

Ingredients:

1 cup of avocado, cubed

1 cup of fresh cherries, pitted

1 whole lime, peeled

1 medium-sized orange, wedged

1 tbsp of honey, raw

Preparation:

Peel the avocado and cut in half. Remove the pit and cut into small cubes. Fill the measuring cup and reserve the rest for later.

Wash the cherries and cut each in half. Remove the pits and set aside.

Peel the lime and cut lengthwise in half. Set aside.

Peel the orange and divide into wedges. Cut each wedge in half and set aside.

Now, combine avocado, cherries, lime, and orange in a juicer and process until well juiced. Transfer to a serving glass and stir in the honey.

Add some crushed ice and serve.

Nutritional information per serving: Kcal: 408, Protein: 6g, Carbs: 74.5g, Fats: 22.5g

28.   Raspberry Apricot Juice

Ingredients:

1 cup of raspberries

1 cup of apricots, sliced

1 medium-sized carrot, sliced

2 whole plums, pitted

1 tbsp of honey, raw

Preparation:

Using a colander, wash the raspberries in under cold running water. Slightly drain and set aside.

Wash the apricots and cut lengthwise in half. Remove the pits and cut into thin slices. Fill the measuring cup and reserve the rest for later.

Wash and peel the carrot. Cut into thin slices and set aside.

Wash the plums and cut in half. Remove the pits and set aside.

Now, combine raspberries, apricots, carrot, and plums in a juicer and process until well juiced.

Transfer to a serving glass and stir in the honey. Add some crushed ice before serving.

Nutritional information per serving: Kcal: 232, Protein: 5.3g, Carbs: 70.9g, Fats: 1.9g

29.   Beet Kiwi Juice

Ingredients:

1 cup of beets, sliced

1 whole kiwi, sliced

1 small apple, cored

1 small pear, cored

¼ tsp of cinnamon, ground

Preparation:

Wash the beets and trim off the green ends. Peel and cut into thin slices. Fill the measuring cup and reserve the rest for some other juice.

Peel the kiwi and cut lengthwise in half. Set aside.

Wash the apple and pear. Remove the core and cut into bite-sized pieces. Set aside.

Now, combine beets, kiwi, apple, and pear in a juicer and process until well juiced. Transfer to a serving glass and stir in the cinnamon. Refrigerate for 15 minutes before serving.

Enjoy!

Nutritional information per serving: Kcal: 211, Protein: 4.2g, Carbs: 65.3g, Fats: 1.1g

30.   Strawberry Avocado Juice

Ingredients:

1 cup of strawberries, chopped

1 cup of avocado, cubed

1 pomegranate seeds

1 cup of cucumber, sliced

1 medium-sized orange, wedged

Preparation:

Wash the strawberries and cut into small pieces. Set aside.

Peel the avocado and cut in half. Remove the pit and cut into cubes. Fill the measuring cup and reserve the rest for later.

Cut the top of the pomegranate fruit using a sharp paring knife. Slice down to each of the white membranes inside of the fruit. Pop the seeds into a measuring cup and set aside.

Wash the cucumber and cut into thin slices. Fill the measuring cup and reserve the rest for later.

Peel the orange and divide into wedges. Chop each wedge in half and set aside.

Now, combine strawberries, avocado, pomegranate, cucumber, and orange in a juicer. Process until well juiced.

Transfer to a serving glass and add some crushed ice before serving.

Nutritional information per serving: Kcal: 335, Protein: 6.6g, Carbs: 53.2g, Fats: 23.5g

31.   Cherry Mango Juice

Ingredients:

1 cup of fresh cherries

1 cup of mango, chunked

1 cup of fresh mint, torn

1 small apple, cored

¼ tsp of ginger, ground

Preparation:

Wash the cherries and cut each in half. Remove the pits and fill the measuring cup. Reserve the rest for some other juice.

Peel the mango and cut into small chunks. Fill the measuring cup and refrigerate the rest for later.

Wash the mint thoroughly under cold running water. Slightly drain and torn with hands. Set aside.

Wash the apple and cut in half. Remove the core and cut into bite-sized pieces. Set aside.

Now, combine cherries, mango, mint, and apple in a juicer and process until juiced. Transfer to a serving glass and stir in the ginger.

Add some ice or refrigerate for 15 minutes before serving.

Nutritional information per serving: Kcal: 262, Protein: 4.3g, Carbs: 75.3g, Fats: 6.6g

32.   Watermelon Grape Juice

Ingredients:

1 cup of watermelon, cubed

1 cup of green grapes

1 whole kiwi, peeled

1 medium-sized pear, chopped

Preparation:

Cut the watermelon lengthwise. Cut one large wedge and peel it. Cut into chunks and fill the measuring cup. Remove the seeds and set aside. Reserve the rest of the melon for some other juices.

Wash the grapes and set aside.

Peel the kiwi and cut lengthwise in half. Set aside.

Wash the pear and remove the core. Cut into bite-sized pieces and set aside.

Now, combine watermelon, grapes, kiwi, and pear in a juicer and process until well juiced.

Transfer to a serving glass and add some crushed ice before serving.

Enjoy!

Nutritional information per serving: Kcal: 216, Protein: 3g, Carbs: 64.5g, Fats: 1.2g

33.   Spinach Kale Juice

Ingredients:

1 cup of fresh spinach, torn

1 cup of fresh kale, torn

1 cup of cabbage, shredded

1 cup of fresh parsley, torn

1 cup of cucumber, sliced

1 cup of avocado, chunked

¼ tsp of turmeric, ground

Preparation:

Combine spinach, kale, and parsley in a large colander. Rinse all under cold running water and slightly drain. Torn with hands and set aside.

Wash the cabbage thoroughly and shred the cabbage. Fill the measuring cup and reserve the rest for later.

Wash the cucumber and cut into thin slices. Set aside.

Peel the avocado and cut in half. Remove the pit and cut into small chunks. Fill the measuring cup and reserve the rest for later.

Now, combine spinach, kale, parsley, cabbage, cucumber, and avocado in a juicer and process until juiced. Transfer to a serving glass and stir in the turmeric.

Refrigerate for 10 minutes and serve.

Nutritional information per serving: Kcal: 272, Protein: 10.9g, Carbs: 33.1g, Fats: 23.5g

34.   Collard Greens Tomato Juice

Ingredients:

1 cup of collard greens, roughly chopped

1 cup of Romaine lettuce, roughly chopped

1 large Roma tomato, chopped

1 medium-sized red bell pepper, chopped

¼ tsp of ginger, ground

Preparation:

Wash collard greens and lettuce thoroughly under cold running water. Roughly chop it and fill the measuring cups. Reserve the rest for later.

Wash the tomato and place it in a small bowl. Cut into small pieces and reserve the tomato juice while cutting.

Wash the bell pepper and cut lengthwise in half. Remove the seeds and cut into small pieces. Set aside.

Now, combine collard greens, lettuce, tomato, and red bell pepper in a juicer and process until well juiced.

Transfer to a serving glass and stir in the ginger. Add some ice or refrigerate for 10 minutes before serving.

Nutritional information per serving: Kcal: 61, Protein: 5.5g, Carbs: 17.7g, Fats: 1.1g

35.   Pear Banana Juice

Ingredients:

1 large pear, chopped

1 large banana, sliced

1 cup of pineapple, chunked

1 whole lemon, peeled

5 cherries, pitted

1 tbsp of honey

Preparation:

Wash the pear and cut in half. Remove the core and cut into bite-sized pieces. Set aside.

Peel the banana and cut into small chunks. Set aside.

Cut the top of a pineapple and peel it using a sharp paring knife. Cut into small chunks and fill the measuring cup. Reserve the rest in a refrigerator.

Peel the lemon and cut lengthwise in half. Set aside.

Wash the cherries and cut each in half. Remove the pits and set aside.

Now, combine pear, banana, pineapple, lemon, and cherries in a juicer and process until juiced. Transfer to a serving glass and stir in the honey.

Refrigerate for 10 minutes before serving.

Nutritional information per serving: Kcal: 374, Protein: 4.3g, Carbs: 109g, Fats: 1.2g

36.   Zucchini Avocado Juice

Ingredients:

1 small zucchini, chopped

1 cup of avocado, chunked

1 cup of mango, chopped

1 whole lime, peeled

1 oz coconut water

1 tsp of fresh mint, finely chopped

Preparation:

Peel the zucchini and cut lengthwise in half. Scrape out the seeds and wash it. Cut into small pieces and set aside.

Peel the avocado and cut in half. Remove the pit and cut into chunks. Set aside.

Wash and peel the mango. Chop into bite-sized pieces and set aside.

Peel the lime and cut lengthwise in half. Set aside.

Now, combine zucchini, avocado, mango, lime, and mint in a juicer and process until juiced. Transfer to a serving glass and stir in the coconut water. Add some crushed ice and serve immediately.

Nutritional information per serving: Kcal: 309, Protein: 5.8g, Carbs: 44.5g, Fats: 22.4g

37.   Pumpkin Apricot Juice

Ingredients:

1 cup of pumpkin, chopped

1 cup of apricots, sliced

2 medium-sized strawberries, chopped

1 small Golden Delicious apple, cored

1 tbsp of liquid honey

Preparation:

Peel the pumpkin and cut in half. Scoop out the seeds using a spoon. Cut one large wedge and peel it. Cut into small chunks and fill the measuring cup. Reserve the rest for later.

Wash the apricots and cut each in half. Remove the pits and thinly slice. Set aside.

Wash the strawberries and cut into bite-sized pieces. Set aside.

Wash the apple and remove the core. Cut into small chunks and set aside.

Now, combine pumpkin, apricots, strawberries, and apple in a juicer and process until juiced. Transfer to a serving glass and stir in the honey.

Add some ice and serve.

Nutritional information per serving: Kcal: 222, Protein: 4g, Carbs: 62.3g, Fats: 1.1g

38.   Fennel Artichoke Juice

Ingredients:

1 cup of fennel, chopped

1 medium-sized artichoke, chopped

1 cup of cucumber, sliced

1 medium-sized carrot, sliced

¼ tsp of turmeric, ground

Preparation:

Wash the fennel bulb and trim off the wilted outer layers. Cut into small pieces and fill the measuring cup. Reserve the rest for some other juice.

Trim off the outer leaves of the artichoke using a sharp paring knife. Wash it and cut into bite-sized pieces. Set aside.

Wash and peel the cucumber. Cut into thin slices and fill the measuring cup. Refrigerate the rest for later.

Wash and peel the carrot. Cut into thin slices and set aside.

Now, combine fennel, artichoke, cucumber, and carrot in a juicer a process until well juiced.

Transfer to a serving glass and stir in the turmeric. Add some ice and serve immediately.

Nutritional information per serving: Kcal: 73, Protein: 6.1g, Carbs: 27.5g, Fats: 0.6g

39.　　Zucchini Tomato Juice

Ingredients:

1 small zucchini, sliced

4 cherry tomatoes, halved

1 medium-sized carrot, sliced

1 small apple, cored

1 whole lime, peeled

Preparation:

Peel the zucchini and cut into thin slices. Set aside.

Wash the cherry tomatoes and cut in half. Set aside.

Wash and peel the carrot. Cut into thin slices and set aside.

Wash the apple and cut lenghtwise in half. Remove the core and cut into bite-sized pieces. Set aside.

Peel the lime and cut lengthwise in half. Set aside.

Now, combine zucchini, tomatoes, carrot, apple, and lime in a juicer and process until well juiced. Transfer to serving glasses and refrigerate before serving.

Nutritional information per serving: Kcal: 119, Protein: 3.4g, Carbs: 35.4g, Fats: 0.9g

40.　Cantaloupe Artichoke Juice

Ingredients:

1 cup of cantaloupe, chopped

1 medium-sized artichoke, chopped

1 medium-sized celery stalk, chopped

1 whole lemon, peeled

1 tbsp of honey

Preparation:

Cut the cantaloupe in half. Scoop out the seeds and cut two wedges and peel them. Chop into chunks and fill the measuring cup. Reserve the rest of the cantaloupe in a refrigerator.

Trim off the outer leaves of the artichoke using a sharp paring knife. Wash it and cut into bite-sized pieces. Set aside.

Wash the celery stalk and cut into bite-sized pieces. Set aside.

Peel the lemon and cut lengthwise in half. Set aside.

Now, combine cantaloupe, artichoke, celery, and lemon in a juicer. Process until juiced. Transfer to a serving glass and stir in the honey.

Add some crushed ice or refrigerate for 15 minutes before serving.

Nutritional information per serving: Kcal: 144, Protein: 6.5g, Carbs: 32.8g, Fats: 0.8g

41.   Pear Cranberry Juice

Ingredients:

2 large pears, chopped

1 cup of cranberries

1 cup of watercress, torn

½ cup of fresh spinach, torn

1 small ginger knob, peeled

Preparation:

Wash the pears and cut in half. Remove the core and cut into bite-sized pieces. Set aside.

Place the cranberries in a colander and rinse thoroughly. Slightly drain and set aside.

Wash watercress and spinach thoroughly under cold running water. Drain and torn with hands. Set aside.

Peel the ginger and set aside.

Now, combine pears, cranberries, watercress, spinach, and ginger in a juicer and process until well juiced. Transfer to a serving glass and stir in some water if you like. However, it is optional.

Refrigerate for 15 minutes before serving.

Enjoy!

Nutritional information per serving: Kcal: 249, Protein: 3.8g, Carbs: 86.1g, Fats: 0.9g

42.   Kiwi Guava Juice

Ingredients:

1 whole kiwi, peeled

1 whole guava, peeled

1 cup of mango, chunked

3 whole plums, pitted

1 oz of water

1 tbsp of liquid honey

Preparation:

Peel the kiwi and cut lengthwise in half. Set aside.

Peel the guava and cut into small pieces. Set aside.

Peel the mango and cut into chunks. Set aside.

Wash the plums and cut in half. Remove the pits and cut into bite-sized pieces. Set aside.

Now, combine kiwi, guava, mango, and plums in a juicer. Process until well juiced. Transfer to a serving glass and stir in the water and honey.

Serve cold.

Nutritional information per serving: Kcal: 286, Protein: 4.9g, Carbs: 65.3g, Fats: 2.1g

43.   Pepper Leek Juice

Ingredients:

1 large red bell pepper, chopped

1 whole leek, chopped

1 small zucchini, chopped

1 medium-sized beet, trimmed and chopped

¼ tsp of salt

Preparation:

Wash the bell pepper and cut lengthwise in half. Remove the seeds and cut into small pieces. Set aside.

Wash the leek and cut into bite-sized pieces. Set aside.

Peel the zucchini and cut into bite-sized pieces. Set aside.

Wash the beets and trim off the green ends. peel and cut into small pieces. Set aside.

Now, combine bell pepper, leek, zucchini, and beet in a juicer. Process until juiced. Transfer to a serving glass and stir in the salt.

Refrigerate for 15 minutes before serving.

Nutritional information per serving: Kcal: 126, Protein: 5.7g, Carbs: 34g, Fats: 1.3g

44.   Sweet Potato Juice

Ingredients:

1 cup of sweet potatoes, chopped

1 cup of asparagus, trimmed

½ cup of green beans, chopped

1 whole lemon, peeled

¼ tsp of turmeric, ground

2 oz of water

Preparation:

Peel the potato and cut into small chunks. Fill the measuring cup and reserve the rest in the refrigerator.

Wash the asparagus and trim off the woody ends. Cut into bite-sized pieces and set aside.

Wash the green beans and cut into small pieces. Set aside.

Peel the lemon and cut lengthwise in half. Set aside.

Now, combine potato, asparagus, green beans, and lemon in a juicer. Process until well juiced. Transfer to a serving glass and stir in the water.

Add some crushed ice and serve immediately.

Nutritional information per serving: Kcal: 135, Protein: 6.1g, Carbs: 39.3g, Fats: 0.5g

45.   Apricot Cauliflower Juice

Ingredients:

2 whole apricots, pitted

1 cauliflower floweret, chopped

1 large carrot, sliced

1 cup of mango, chunked

1 cup of Swiss chard

¼ tsp of ginger, ground

Preparation:

Wash the apricots and cut lengthwise in half. Remove the pits and cut into small pieces. Set aside.

Rinse the cauliflower and roughly chop it. Set aside.

Wash and peel the carrot. Cut into thin slices and set aside.

Wash the mango and cut into small chunks. Fill the measuring cup and reserve the rest for later.

Wash the Swiss chard under cold running water. Slightly drain and roughly chop it. Set aside.

Now, combine apricots, cauliflower, carrot, mango, and Swiss chard in a juicer and process until well juiced.

Transfer to a serving glass and stir in the water and ginger. Add some ice and serve immediately.

Nutritional information per serving: Kcal: 149, Protein: 4.4g, Carbs: 42.5g, Fats: 1.3g

46.   Grapefruit Melon Juice

Ingredients:

1 whole grapefruit, wedged

1 honeydew melon wedge, peeled

1 large banana, sliced

1 whole lime, peeled

1 small orange, wedged

1 tbsp of liquid honey

Preparation:

Peel the grapefruit and divide into wedges. Cut each wedge in half and set aside.

Cut one large honeydew melon wedge and peel it. Remove the seeds and cut into bite-sized pieces. Set aside.

Peel the banana and cut into thin slices. Set aside.

Peel the lime and cut lengthwise in half. Set aside.

Peel the orange and divide into wedges. Cut each wedge in half and set aside.

Now, combine grapefruit, melon, banana, lime, and orange in a juicer and process until juiced.

Transfer to a serving glass and add some ice before serving.

Enjoy!

Nutritional information per serving: Kcal: 281, Protein: 5.2g, Carbs: 83.6g, Fats: 1.2g

47. Fennel Avocado Juice

Ingredients:

1 cup of fennel, chopped

1 cup of avocado, chunked

1 small Granny Smith's apple, chopped

1 cup of cucumber, sliced

¼ tsp of ginger, ground

Preparation:

Wash the fennel bulb and trim off the wilted outer layers. Cut into small chunks and fill the measuring cup. Reserve the rest in the refrigerator.

Peel the avocado and cut in half. Remove the pit and cut into small chunks. Fill the measuring cup and reserve the rest for later.

Wash the apple and remove the core. Cut into bite-sized pieces and set aside.

Wash the cucumber and cut into thin slices. Fill the measuring cup and reserve the rest in the refrigerator. Set aside.

121 Complete Weight Gaining Shake and Meal Recipes to Get Bigger and Stronger

Now, combine fennel, avocado, apple, and cucumber in a juicer and process until juiced. Transfer to a serving glass and stir in the ginger.

Add some ice before serving.

Nutritional information per serving: Kcal: 286, Protein: 5g, Carbs: 40.3g, Fats: 21.9g

48.   Blackberry Banana Juice

Ingredients:

1 cup of blackberries

1 large banana, sliced

1 whole beet, trimmed

1 small green apple, chopped

¼ tsp of cinnamon, ground

Preparation:

Place the blackberries in a colander and rinse well under cold running water. Slightly drain and set aside.

Peel the banana and cut into thin slices. Set aside.

Wash the beet and trim off the green ends. Slightly peel and cut into small pieces. Set aside.

Wash the apple and cut in half. Remove the core and cut into bite-sized pieces. Set aside.

Now, combine blackberries, banana, beet, and apple in a juicer and process until well juiced. Transfer to a serving glass and stir in the cinnamon.

Refrigerate for 15 minutes before serving.

Nutritional information per serving: Kcal: 233, Protein: 5.4g, Carbs: 72.3g, Fats: 1.6g

49.   Orange Pomegranate Juice

Ingredients:

1 medium-sized orange, peeled

1 cup of pomegranate seeds

1 small pear, chopped

1 small zucchini, chopped

1 cup of fresh mint, torn

1 tbsp of liquid honey

Preparation:

Peel the orange and divide into wedges. Cut each wedge in half and set aside.

Cut the top of the pomegranate fruit using a sharp paring knife. Slice down to each of the white membranes inside of the fruit. Pop the seeds into a measuring cup and set aside.

Wash the pear and cut in half. Remove the core and cut into bite-sized pieces. Set aside.

Peel the zucchini and cut into small chunks. Set aside.

Rinse the mint under cold running water using a colander. Slightly drain and torn with hands. Set aside.

Now, combine orange, pomegranate seeds, pear, zucchini, and mint in a juicer and process until juiced. Transfer to a serving glass and stir in the honey.

Add some crushed ice and serve immediately.

Nutritional information per serving: Kcal: 259, Protein: 5.6g, Carbs: 61.6g, Fats: 2.1g

50.   Green Sweet Potato Juice

Ingredients:

1 cup of sweet potatoes, chopped

1 cup of turnip greens, torn

1 cup of fresh kale, torn

1 cup of fresh parsley, torn

1 cup of avocado, chunked

1 small green apple, chopped

¼ tsp of ginger, ground

1 tbsp of liquid honey

1 oz of water

Preparation:

Peel the potato and wash it. Cut into small chunks and fill the measuring cup. Reserve the rest in the refrigerator.

Combine turnip greens, kale, and parsley in a large colander. Rinse thoroughly under cold running water. Slightly drain and torn all with hands. Set aside.

Peel the avocado and cut lengthwise in half. Remove the pit and cut into chunks and fill the measuring cup. Reserve the rest for later. Set aside.

Wash the apple and cut in half. Remove the core and cut into bite-sized pieces. Set aside.

Now, combine sweet potato, turnip greens, kale, parsley, avocado, and apple in a juicer and process until juiced. Transfer to a serving glass and stir in the ginger, honey, and water.

Refrigerate for 15 minutes before serving.

Enjoy!

Nutritional information per serving: Kcal: 474, Protein: 11.1g, Carbs: 72.7g, Fats: 23.6g

51.   Bean Broccoli Juice

Ingredients:

1 cup of green beans, chopped

1 cup of fresh broccoli, chopped

1 cup of cucumber, sliced

1 cup of mustard greens, torn

1 cup of yam, chopped

1 small ginger knob, peeled

2 oz of water

Preparation:

Wash the green beans and cut into small pieces. Set aside.

Wash the broccoli and cut into bite-sized pieces. Set aside.

Wash the cucumber and cut into thin slices. Fill the measuring cup and reserve the rest for later.

Rinse the mustard greens thoroughly under cold running water. Torn with hands and set aside.

Peel the yam and cut into chunks. Fill the measuring cup and reserve the rest for later.

Peel the ginger knob and set aside.

Now, combine green beans, broccoli, cucumber, mustard greens, yam, and ginger in a juicer and process until juiced.

Transfer to a serving glass and stir in the water.

Add some ice and serve immediately.

Nutritional information per serving: Kcal: 213, Protein: 7.9g, Carbs: 57.2g, Fats: 1.1g

52.   Blueberry Cherry Juice

Ingredients:

1 cup of blueberries

1 cup of cherries, pitted

1 cup of black grapes

1 small blood orange, wedged

¼ tsp of cinnamon, ground

Preparation:

Combine blueberries and grapes in a colander and wash under cold running water. Slightly drain and set aside.

Wash the cherries and cut each in half. Remove the pits and set aside.

Peel the orange and divide into wedges. Cut each wedge in half and set aside.

Now, combine blueberries, cherries, grapes, and orange in a juicer and process until juiced.

Transfer to a serving glass and stir in the cinnamon.

Add some ice and serve immediately.

Nutritional information per serving: Kcal: 249, Protein: 4.2g, Carbs: 73.2g, Fats: 1.2g

ADDITIONAL TITLES FROM THIS AUTHOR

70 Effective Meal Recipes to Prevent and Solve Being Overweight: Burn Fat Fast by Using Proper Dieting and Smart Nutrition

By

Joe Correa CSN

48 Acne Solving Meal Recipes: The Fast and Natural Path to Fixing Your Acne Problems in Less Than 10 Days!

By

Joe Correa CSN

41 Alzheimer's Preventing Meal Recipes: Reduce or Eliminate Your Alzheimer's Condition in 30 Days or Less!

By

Joe Correa CSN

70 Effective Breast Cancer Meal Recipes: Prevent and Fight Breast Cancer with Smart Nutrition and Powerful Foods

By

Joe Correa CSN

www.ingramcontent.com/pod-product-compliance
Lightning Source LLC
Chambersburg PA
CBHW030242030426
42336CB00009B/217